What people are saying about...

COOPERATIVE WELLNESS

"I couldn't put it down! If you read *Cooperative Wellness* with an open mind and heart, you'll receive the invaluable benefit of Dr. Rall's unwavering commitment to truth. His gift of communicating this passion to countless patients with bold encouragement and common-sense application shines through in this book. I am grateful to Dr. Rall for inspiring me to trust more deeply and experience more fully the body's God-given power to heal — and am so glad that others can share in this information as well. *Cooperative Wellness* ignites the inner courage needed to choose personal transformation as the only way to revolutionize healthcare for everyone."

Emily French | Self-Health Enthusiast

"When looking at our society as a whole, we either do not want to believe there is a problem with our current healthcare system or we are aware of the problem but do not know what we can do to fix it. In this book, Dr. Rall raises critical questions about why our healthcare model is flawed and shows exactly what you can do to change it. Whether you are an employee who wants change or an employer who wants to offer a true solution to your employees, *Cooperative Wellness* is for you."

Daniel & Dr. Kimberly Huck | Owners of American Row House Gyms

"My first foray into corporate wellness was in 1981. Since then, the personal state of health in the USA has only dramatically worsened. It just isn't working because health is a personal choice. Cooperation, however, offers the best and most reasonable hope for our sustainable well-being. Dr. Rall paints a vibrant rationale and philosophy grounded in realism. Read *Cooperative Wellness!* He makes a common-sense argument for living life on purpose, which is best realized when we're robustly cooperating in our health."

**Kevin W. McCarthy | Author, *The On-Purpose Person*
and *The On-Purpose Business Person***

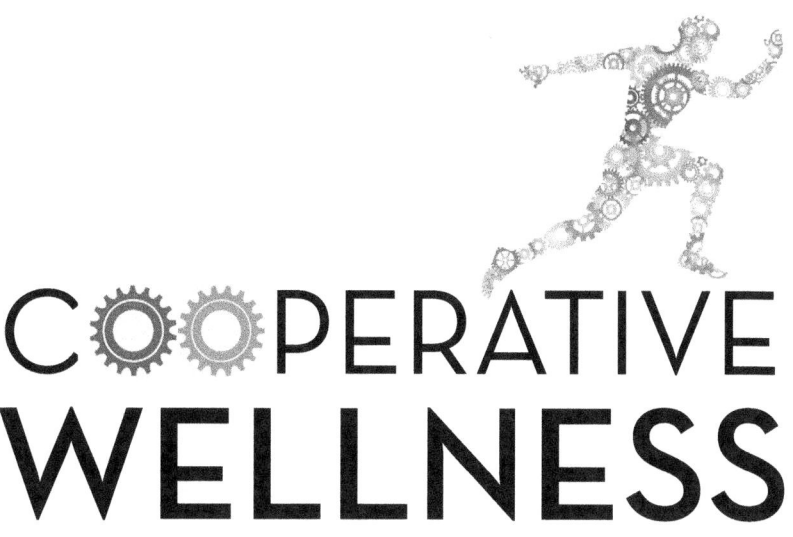

C⚙⚙PERATIVE WELLNESS

How to Achieve Wellness
and Be Part of the Healthcare Solution

(It's Easier Than You Think!)

Dr. Ben Rall

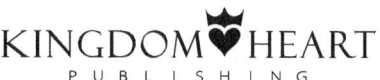

KINGDOM♥HEART
PUBLISHING

To those who have yet to know
where true health comes from.

ACKNOWLEDGMENTS

I would like to acknowledge those trailblazers who have gone before me. Without people who were willing to believe there must be a better way to manage health, we would not be able to have these conversations. These revolutionaries include: Dr. Reggie Gold, Dr. Fred Barge, Dr. Clarence Gonstead, Dr. DD Palmer, and Dr. BJ Palmer.

To my countless colleagues, but specifically Dr. Dan Sullivan, who continues to help me sharpen my ax.

To Dr. Pete Camiolo who brings me back to the source.

To Junior and Tama Davis for being caring enough about people to make a difference.

To Anj Marie Riffel of Kingdom Heart Publishing for editing and design and to Michelle C. Booth for proofreading.

To Pastor David Uth for showing me the real value of all God's people.

To my wife Megan and children who have taken this journey together, and have been willing to go wherever this road takes us.

To all my patients past, present, and future. Thank you for teaching me every day where the greatest doctor in the world lives…inside you!

To my Lord and Savior, Jesus Christ.

ABOUT THE AUTHOR

Dr. Ben Rall was born and raised in the great state of South Dakota. He lives in Orlando, Florida, with his wife, Megan, and two children, Jack and Grace. Dr. Rall owned and operated one of the largest chiropractic and wellness clinics in the United States, and currently helps individuals and organizations apply a vitalistic model of healthcare to their lives.

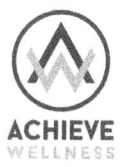

ACHIEVE
WELLNESS

www.achievewellness.clinic
info@achievewellness.clinic

TABLE OF CONTENTS

FOREWORD

The Elegance of Simplicity

By Christopher Labrecque

"No man will make a great leader who wants to do it all himself, or to get all the credit for doing it."
— Andrew Carnegie

In the time that I have known Dr. Ben Rall, it's been quite an education for me. The two of us were brought together in a work environment, and have since packed a serious amount of challenging, arguing, developing, and finally—trusting—into that short time period.

While we still disagree on certain matters (as most people do), what we have is a much-needed level of respect and trust that is fundamental to working together in a challenging environment. Like two pilots in an unexpected nosedive, we must trust and respect one another in order to overcome the crisis at hand. There is so little of this type of mutual respect and cooperation these days, particularly in areas of heated debate, and that only exacerbates the problem.

In my 25 professional years, I've never worked with anyone remotely like Dr. Rall, and that's a good thing. I write that with a wink and a smile, but what I really mean is that I needed all those years to prepare for the journey that he and I were going to embark on together.

After our first meeting, I recall thinking to myself, "I pray this man's motives are solid." You see, I'd witnessed energy and enthusiasm like his many times before, but it always turned out to be self-serving. Now having worked with Dr. Rall, I see that's not so, and I am greatly relieved.

To overcome the healthcare challenge our nation faces, we need to engineer an environment in which the motives between the complementing—not competing—parties are aligned. No one man, no one institution, no one industry stands to do this alone. It requires a concerted effort in which the end user/patient remains at the center of an intense level of education, resourcing, and simplification. Then, and only then, do we have a chance to overcome the greatest challenge of our generation.

The blurred lines between stakeholders is where we need to reside for now, challenging each other, but respectfully so. It is in this intersecting space that breakthroughs occur. The book you hold in your hands was written upon this cusp of breakthrough, and it is here that readers of *Cooperative Wellness* have much to gain.

I think Dr. Rall can remain confident that he has provided insights to simple—yet foundational—solutions, that can in turn simplify the broader, more complex problems of healthcare. And in doing so, he has challenged the varied interests that may collide on these matters to work cooperatively, respectfully, and successfully together.

The healthcare crisis can and will be overcome; it is not insurmountable. As Dr. Rall has presented in this text, the elegance of the solution oftentimes remains in its simplicity.

Christopher Labrecque is managing partner of Employee Benefits Group, IOA.

PREFACE

Why I Wrote This Book

"The quality of your life is based upon the quality of the questions you ask." — Dr. John Demartini

I have two children. They have probably asked, "Why?" thousands of times. As any parent knows, this incessant questioning can become frustrating, but my kids are simply engaging in one of life's most profound pursuits.

Asking why is the catalyst to understanding. It connects us to the deeper quest of defining our purpose, which is the essence of life. It is the most fundamental of questions, and the very best place to begin when it comes to our health.

To that end, this book will try to answer a few whys in regard to our nation's poor state of health and show how it's supported by a broken health system. Even more so, I hope this book will inspire you to begin asking why, if you're not already.

As with any large problem, finding a solution can seem over-whelming. Where do you even begin? I decided to begin from my current point of reference, as a doctor who has seen firsthand the benefits of a vitalistic (also known as holistic or natural) approach to medicine—as someone who understands and views the body as a self-healing, self-regulating organism. I also decided to begin by focusing on my current sphere of influence, the people I work with every day.

You can do the same.

Whether you're an employer or an employee, we all have a purpose. We all fill a role and serve a need. We're here for a reason. One of the most untapped resources in terms of a person's value—whether to our families, our workplace, or our world—is acknowledgment of purpose.

Helping people find the vitality, health, and wellness they need to fully reach their purpose is a very noble and honorable role you can play.

How can you do this?

By becoming part of the solution. At a high-level, by being an employer that truly cares about the well-being and best interests of your employees. Or by being an employee that engages in the pursuit of improved healthcare for yourself and the betterment of those around you.

I wrote this book to help. I wrote it for you, your family, your colleagues, and for the vast majority of Americans who receive their healthcare under the auspices of company-managed health insurance coverage.

As a country, we have been misled for too long about why we receive care the way we do. It's time for all of us to realize what's at stake, as well as the role we each play in our current health predicament.

That's why I'm advocating for a shift from that tired idea of corporate wellness to a new model of cooperative wellness. It's important to note that while cooperation requires parts working together as a greater whole, it doesn't necessarily happen easily or smoothly.

As with the non-violent protests associated with many historical movements, cooperative does not mean passive. The conversion to cooperative wellness will be dramatic and powerful, and it won't happen without intentional effort.

Cooperative wellness has many layers. We need to cooperate with our bodies. And we need to cooperate with each other. Together, we really can achieve wellness. We can get our families, our companies, and our nation on the road to better health and investing in a healthcare system that actually works to help people.

Perhaps the best news of all is that the solution is easier than you think.

INTRODUCTION
Achieving Wellness Is Easier Than You Think

"As a human being, you have no choice about the fact that you need a philosophy. Your only choice is whether you define your philosophy by a conscious, rational, disciplined process of thought and scrupulously logical deliberation — or let your subconscious accumulate a junk heap of unwarranted conclusions, false generalizations, undefined contradictions, undigested slogans, unidentified wishes, doubts, and fears, thrown together by chance, but integrated by your subconscious into a kind of mongrel philosophy and fused into a single, solid weight: self-doubt, like a ball and chain in the place where your mind's wings should have grown."
— Ayn Rand and Leonard Peikoff

The human body is a marvel. Its mechanisms of internal cooperation display a depth and complexity beyond our understanding. This is why conventional approaches to repairing our health fall short—rather than augmenting the body's natural cooperation with itself, we try to directly manipulate one small part of the system and often disrupt the rest in our ignorance.

This is the real reason for all those side effects listed in drug commercials—if you can tell me the difference between a desired effect and a side effect, beyond whether the drug's inventor would want it to occur or not, I'd love to hear it.

When you attempt to manipulate one part of the body without fully understanding its cooperative relationship with the other parts, you are likely to do more harm than good.

A 2009 study published in the *Journal of the American Medical Association* by Charles Kilo and Eric Larson, both MDs, found that despite spending trillions of dollars on healthcare each year, the benefits that the U.S. healthcare system currently delivers may not outweigh the aggregate harm it causes.[1]

We currently spend 17 percent of our Gross Domestic Product (GDP)—$3 trillion—on healthcare as a nation. Kilo and Larson's data suggests we might have been better off spending nothing at all than to have invested what we have in drugs, surgeries, and other interventions whose short-term effects seem like a gamble at best and long-term effects remain to be seen.

It's an astonishing finding, the equivalent of wondering whether we might have had fewer fires and robberies if we'd never bothered hiring police officers or firefighters. It seems unimaginable, but the very fact that we have to question whether our healthcare system has any net value is sobering.

All of this is to convey the magnitude and ramifications of this discussion of cooperation. It's about much more than "getting along"—as a matter of fact, getting along isn't necessarily cooperating. Putting up with a broken, sick, dangerous system to avoid rocking the boat is not cooperating, it's enabling.

When we choose to mask our symptoms, we are actually giving the underlying causes the opportunity to proliferate. For example, if my blood pressure is high because of lifestyle choices and my doctor prescribes medication to artificially lower it, we are allowing the disease to progress.

The current medical model is so ingrained in our culture, anything else is viewed as irresponsible, but we've got it backward. Moving toward a cooperative model of healthcare will require nothing short of a revolution. However, it can—and should—be a peaceful and productive one, a revolution of clarity and understanding to vanquish an unsustainable, profit-driven conglomerate that's trafficking in half-truths and outright deception.

After working with thousands of patients in the health and wellness space—from newborn babies to Olympic athletes to the elderly—several things have become apparent.

For one, I've spotted some common barriers that prevent people from getting the best possible care for themselves and their families. Most of the objections my patients would raise to any particular course of action boil down to not having enough time.

COMMON HEALTH OBSTACLES:
1. I don't have time to cook healthy food.
2. I don't have time to exercise.
3. I don't have time for this treatment program right now.

This is part of the reason we need to reimagine workplace wellness. In round numbers, people spend one-third of their day at the office and one-third sleeping, which only leaves one-third for anything else, including exercise. Especially for people with sedentary jobs, it makes sense to better integrate healthcare efforts into our workday to the greatest extent possible. (No, I'm not talking about treadmill desks, although that wouldn't hurt.)

Another common hurdle to receiving effective treatment is money. I've lost count of the number of times I've heard a variation on the following: "Doc, I really need your help, but I just don't think I can afford it." In reality, you can't afford *not* to regain your health. What people are really saying is, "I won't do this if it's not covered by insurance." In our current distorted thinking about healthcare, we'd rather get the wrong treatment at the right price.

These experiences led me on a journey. Rather than let the faulty incentives of the health insurance system warp my standards of care, I transitioned to a 100-percent cash practice, while devoting a significant amount of my time to community and corporate education efforts focused on prevention. I started working with school districts, large and small companies, churches, and nonprofits to create wellness programs that work for them. True health begins with knowledge, so helping others understand and take ownership of their own health was the most effective way I could make change happen.

The success of this patient-centered wellness model grew our clinic into one of the largest of its kind in the United States. I was also able to spend time in other countries, helping to open wellness clinics and deliver education on the subjects covered in these pages.

From there, I had the opportunity to help oversee one of the largest networks of wellness centers in North America. I helped develop programs and training for doctors and patients to have the resources and support they needed in an easy, effective, and affordable model. While I knew the problem was larger than this nationwide network of wellness centers could address, I held out hope that a little political goodwill on both sides of the aisle might lead to legislation to tackle the fundamental problems.

Eventually however, I came to accept that these issues will not be solved in Washington. To really make a change, I knew I had to work from a grassroots perspective and get directly involved in the corporate model. After all, that's where most of us get our healthcare: our day jobs. I needed to partner with employers to help them improve their bottom line and overall business by dramatically improving the health of their employees (not to mention their own health as well).

That's exactly what I do now: help employers give their employees effective wellness options and help employees understand the true foundations of healthy living.

Whether you're a healthcare provider or advocate, frontline employee, manager, head of your company's benefits department, or CEO of a Fortune 500 corporation, the question of how companies can better foster the health and wellness of their employees affects you, your colleagues, and your family.

What follows is an argument—backed by hard science and much experience—for the changes both individuals and organizations can make today to achieve a healthier workplace and a healthier nation for all of us.

CHAPTER ONE

Why Our Healthcare System Isn't Working

"The significant problems we face cannot be solved at the same level of thinking we were at when we created them."
— Albert Einstein

Given our health-crazed culture, you'd think we'd be well on our way to a healthy society. But in spite of an abundance of bike trails, gyms, and natural food stores, America's love of couches, TV, and fast-food is still alive and well.

The same is true in our workplaces. When you think about corporate wellness done right, your mind probably goes to the cutting-edge tech companies who have both the money and incentive to treat employees like royalty. After all, competition for the best and brightest talent is fierce.

This new gold standard of corporate wellness usually includes coveted benefits such as free yoga, posh fitness facilities, free organic lunches in the cafeteria, subsidized on-site massage, and so on—along with insurance plans offering broad coverage and low premiums. Sounds pretty good, right?

The uncomfortable truth is that these plush extras might tip the scales in luring on-the-fence recruits, but they don't move the needle when it comes to employee health outcomes. While intentions may vary among corporations, they largely have the same approach of throwing money at "wellness," possibly hoping something sticks, and proud of the effort either way. But if employees aren't any healthier for it, these expensive extras are the equivalent of a nicer bed for your ambulance ride.

What's going wrong? Why aren't these wellness-pampered employees getting healthier?

For one thing, most of these corporate wellness programs—from Employee Assistance Programs (EAPs) to free yoga classes—are chronically underutilized. What's more, anyone who legitimately thinks offering a few hours of on-site massage every now and then will impact healthcare outcomes is sadly deceived at best, but more likely indifferent.

Some call this approach "Jacuzzi wellness." It might feel good — assuming anyone bothers to use it — but it costs the company a bundle and makes no measurable impact on employee health.

By the way, the money spent on these little-used luxuries comes out of the budget that could go toward benefits that might actually, you know, *benefit* people.

I recently asked a corporate wellness director at one of these large tech companies about their famously comprehensive array of benefits and couldn't believe what he told me.

"I have a pretty good gig," he said. "I have what amounts to a blank check to pay for these programs. In our industry, it's simply expected to offer these perks. We even have a beautiful on-site gym with keycard access."

Then he added, "Thanks to the keycards, we can easily see how few of our employees actually go inside."

My heart sank. Must be nice not to be held accountable for outcomes, eh?

I responded, "But shouldn't the point of the company's wellness efforts be focused on actually keeping the employees healthier?"

"I would strongly encourage you," he replied, "not to tie corporate wellness to the healthcare benefits bottom line."

At that point, I almost dropped the phone.

You might think I'm overreacting. After all, who doesn't like a free massage now and then? If only it were so simple.

In the smaller sense, programs with the stated purpose of making employees healthier have become thinly veiled recruitment tools, comfy perks along the lines of access to a company car. Ironically, the very same companies that offer health luxuries also offer unlimited fountain soda, alcohol on-tap, sleep pods, and video-game suites.

In the larger sense, these pseudo-wellness efforts breed cynicism toward the clinically and economically proven effectiveness of a holistic wellness approach. True wellness programs (more on this later) have been shown time and again to improve employee health outcomes and reduce the cost of healthcare across the board—yet they are nowhere to be seen at most large U.S. companies.

To be fair, the problem can be hard to see. It's very easy for both employers and employees to lose sight of the true bottom-line costs of healthcare—and that is by design. Health insurance companies want Americans to believe that corporate-sponsored healthcare doesn't cost much. They go to great lengths to ensure that the system veils the black-and-white costs to employees, employers, and government.

The truth is that rising healthcare costs in the United States are taking an increasingly disastrous toll on employee paychecks, company profitability, and the national economy — with no end in sight.

The only possible remedy to the situation is a true wellness-oriented approach to healthcare. It can begin simply through the intentionality and cooperation of employees and employers. Hopefully, health insurance providers and government entities will follow suit and embrace this vision as well.

REDEFINING WELLNESS

A great first step for companies would be to call a perk a perk. It's destructive when we mislabel employee perks as "wellness programs." People walk away thinking wellness doesn't work. (It does.)

The next myth to debunk is that cheaper is better. I'm not arguing for ways to somehow squeeze costs out of the current system. Cheaper drugs and cheaper MRIs would not make us one bit healthier as a country. In fact, if every single component of our healthcare system suddenly became free tomorrow, evidence shows that this would not make us healthier at all.

So what can be done?

While multinational drug companies may try to muddy the waters, we have solid science to answer the question. What actually makes people healthier? It has nothing to do with smart drugs, robot surgeons, or miracle therapies.

Researchers and practitioners are well aware of inexpensive, easy interventions that — if implemented throughout the healthcare system — could have a dramatic effect on the health of our nation, saving trillions in the long-term.

Instead of working toward true wellness, we continue to naively float down the river of tradition, believing that interventions like offering free annual medical screenings are the ticket to employee health.

Consider this typical scenario: An employee's blood pressure registers high at the company health fair. The nurse offers rote advice about vegetables and exercise and refers the employee to a physician who prescribes a new, expensive medication. The employee continues to lead the same lifestyle that likely caused the problem in the first place, and now we've added a host of side-effects from the medication to the picture (with potential long-term hazards yet to be discovered).

There are effective holistic alternatives to the typical drug-centered treatment protocols that mostly mask the symptom without addressing the cause. However, if (a) doctors don't consider these alternatives, (b) patients aren't made aware of them, and (c) insurance providers don't incentivize a holistic-first approach, it is highly unlikely that any party will reap the benefits of actually solving the problem.

If high blood pressure is largely a symptom of an unhealthy life-style, the solution should focus on helping the employee improve that lifestyle, not on artificially lowering the blood pressure with a drug. It's the equivalent of turning off the fire alarm in a burning building instead of grabbing a bucket.

As long as this is our general approach to health and wellness, we will not see a reduction in costs or an improvement in outcomes.

High cholesterol is another common health-fair diagnosis. Did you know as much as 90 percent of cholesterol is made by your body? If you see the body as a sophisticated and intelligent system, your assumption will be that it must make cholesterol for a reason. If, on the other hand, you think of the body as a haphazard clunker, you're more likely to think that "high" cholesterol should be "fixed" with a drug. In truth, cholesterol is critical to many functions; it is in every single cell of your body. Without cholesterol, you would be dead.

Instead of signing up for a lifetime of Lipitor, this might be worth some investigation. Why is the cholesterol high? Does lowering cholesterol levels with a drug actually make a person healthier? Research suggests that medicating for high cholesterol has not helped change health outcomes in any significant way.[2] However, pharmaceutical companies would rather not market such discoveries regarding lucrative drugs.

A BETTER WAY

By perpetuating a broken system, many companies are often unwittingly doing more harm to their employees than good through misguided healthcare efforts.

But not everyone gets it wrong. In fact, some lesser-known companies are getting serious results in wellness, measured both in terms of employee health and in cost savings.

One such company bucking the prevailing model is Rosen Hotels & Resorts, a Florida-based chain. Rosen has found a way to integrate wellness by bringing a substantial portion of employee healthcare in-house.

By offering in-house healthcare, Rosen Hotels & Resorts saves millions in premiums each year, has improved employee retention, and has increased productivity with healthier employees.

Rosen employees have access to on-campus physicians for little-to-no fee and can schedule visits during work hours. They also enjoy access to wellness resources, such as smoking cessation programs, which are integrated directly into the daily routines of the workplace.

Although an in-house clinic may seem extreme, the results are impressive. Between 1991 and 2014, Rosen Hotels & Resorts saved more than $225 million on employee and dependent healthcare costs, relative to the traditional fully insured model—with a staggering 8:1 return on investment. Their turnover rate was about 12 percent in 2013, which is significantly lower than the U.S. Bureau of Labor and Statistics' estimated average of 62.6 percent for the hospitality industry.[3]

Harris Rosen has done an amazing job of balancing the health of his employees with the health of his bottom line. He realized that Jacuzzi wellness would only increase his costs and become an entitlement, rather than an incentive for employees to take charge of their own health. By looking at the needs of his employees and the drivers in healthcare costs, he identified effective solutions for his employees and has beaten the system at its own game.

Rosen has presented a concept in which every company with less than 150 employees could provide health insurance in exchange for a federal tax credit of about $4,000 per person. A traditional tax deduction would be available for those over the 150-person limit. It has been estimated that the U.S. could save more than $1 trillion yearly if all companies followed the Rosen approach.

Rosen's example is encouraging, but there's still a lot of fruit on the tree waiting to be picked. We need to get the word out that there's a better way available—one that's producing real results for trailblazing companies like Rosen.

INSURANCE ISN'T FREE

When you pull back the curtain on the operation of today's medical-industrial complex, you find some disturbing realities.

First, the employer generally has a relationship with an insurance broker that solicits bids from insurers and makes a recommendation. The employer then determines what percentage of that cost to shoulder (based on federal regulation) and the rest is deducted from employee paychecks.

The broker generally receives a percentage of the gross sale of the insurance—it's the fox guarding the henhouse. So one of the largest line items on a company's financial statement is being outsourced to a party whose interests are not aligned with the employer, much less the employees.

Now the employees are spending a fair bit each month for insurance and decide they might as well use it. After all, you wouldn't want that insurance to "go to waste." This is where things really fall apart.

The consumer mindset of using the healthcare system simply because you're paying for it causes no end of harm. When people meet their deductible for the year, some treat it as an opportunity for a medical shopping spree.

Beyond the obvious problem of binging on costly and unnecessary interventions, what many don't understand is that they still end up paying for it. In fact, *all* employees will pay for it on the next renewal when the insurer hikes its rates.

Can you blame people? We're told by experts in the media that "smart people go to the doctor." Our friends, relatives, and coworkers tell us we should "have that checked out." Concerned about our health, we go, we get tests, we follow recommendations for drugs and get more tests. Before we know it, we've met our deductible, so heck, why not get a couple more tests done, get another prescription, maybe see a specialist about some nagging complaint? At the end of the year, the insurance company says, "Look how many people are using the insurance! How are we going to pay for this?" And up go the rates.

The other piece of this is that most people never see the actual costs of treatment. "Transparent medical costs" is an oxymoron. If people were told the true costs associated with certain tests or procedures beforehand, they would think twice about having them done. The numbers for some protocols are unconscionable relative to their significance—from the $30 hospital aspirin to getting an MRI since your insurance "covers" it when a much cheaper x-ray would have sufficed. If employees had to pay out of their own pockets, you can be sure they would be more inclined to ask real questions and seek out other solutions to their health problems.

When employees have more skin in the game — higher deductibles, health savings accounts, and so on — they use the system less, which reduces overall costs.

It's time to get in the game. We must understand our roles as employees and employers in managing healthcare costs. We must demand transparency. We must be willing to take our money elsewhere.

In 2015, the average annual cost-per-person for healthcare was estimated to hit $10,000, according to Forbes.[4] If that money were placed directly in the hands of consumers, you would see things change fast. People would spend more judiciously. Healthcare providers would need to attract patients with a value-based plan. Providers have no need to do that now because the money is in the hands of insurance companies—publicly traded, profit-driven companies. This arrangement is not in the best interests of employees nor employers, yet it continues unabated.

To my mind, our healthcare situation is insane. No other industry that I know of operates like this. The results of our misguided approach are all around us—in the abysmal health outcomes that have become common across the country, and in the ballooning economic crisis spurred by health costs. We can do better. We must.

Once the light bulb goes on, you can never see the system in the same way again. It becomes obvious that the best way out of this mess lies in educating employers and employees about the resources they need to disengage from the system. Every dollar spent by your company on teaching people how to effectively use and require less medical care becomes a good investment. Contracting with holistic healthcare providers who can work directly with employees begins to seem like the incredible bargain it really is.

The first step is simply opening our eyes and our minds to what's really going on and then taking personal responsibility.

ADOPTING A GROWTH MINDSET

When facing serious health problems, we often want to blame someone other than the person in the mirror. Although the root cause isn't always clear-cut, it's essential to take ownership of your own health—a victim mindset assumes you cannot change your circumstances.

Stanford psychology professor Carol Dweck has done groundbreaking research on the impact of different mindsets on personal growth.[5]

> If you have a "fixed" mindset, you attribute your situation to external circumstances and are far less likely to invest sustained effort in changing them. If you have a "growth" mindset, you see your situation as something you can influence with effort.

This is a powerful concept as it relates to health. A fixed mindset toward your own health isn't just limiting—it can be deadly.

Here are a few classic examples of a fixed mindset as it relates to health:

- Well my whole family is obese, so I guess I just have the obesity gene.

- Severe headaches are simply part of the stress of a busy executive's life.

- Blood pressure is just one of those things that gets worse with age. Nothing to be done about it.

In reality, while they may be influenced by stress, genetics, and age—obesity, headaches, and high blood pressure are fundamentally symptoms of poor lifestyle choices. Different choices yield different outcomes. Until we adopt a growth mindset toward our own health, we are doomed to continue the same behaviors that caused these problems in the first place.

Consider the common cold. Most anyone over the age of six who gets a cold feels confident that they will get completely better. Same goes for the flu. You may feel terrible, but experience tells you that in a few days it'll be as though nothing ever happened. Amazing, right? A drug doesn't do that—your body does. Sure, you could take some over-the-counter drugs (with effects both seen and unseen) to dry up your runny nose, but your body will heal either way. You could run to the local urgent care clinic, get some tests done, and get a prescription for your cough, but you'll still recover in the same amount of time. The only difference is the hundreds, even thousands, of dollars this approach will cost your insurance plan (and ultimately, you).

What many people don't realize is that the vast majority of healing happens naturally inside your body, unseen and unfelt at the cellular level. This healing is far more amazing than the muted impact of a decongestant on a stuffy nose, but since you don't experience its effect directly, it's easy to take your body's intrinsic healing powers for granted. Even as you sit reading this book, trillions of cells in your body are busily repairing themselves. Cancer cells are being destroyed, your liver and lungs and heart are being repaired and rebuilt, and on and on. If you learn to appreciate this symphony of healing, you can begin to give it the proper respect.

Considering how we treat ourselves, our society should be even sicker than we are. Our bodies do an astonishingly good job keeping us going, no matter what we throw at them. Think of your body like a plant that grows fine on its own as long as it has soil, water, light, and nutrients. If it's wilting, you don't say, "I bet that ficus needs Prozac!" You look at what the plant innately needs and try to provide it. This is the mindset we need to adopt toward our bodies.

When we view our health from this informed perspective, realizing that natural, holistic lifestyle changes are the best way to help the body heal itself, the problems with the current medical approach become glaring.

Today, anyone (without a vested interest) will admit that the pharmaceutical-driven model of treatment has not delivered the health outcomes it has promised—and continues to promise. According to *The Washington Post,* pharmaceutical companies spent $4.5 billion on prescription drug ads in 2014 alone.[6] We have gone too far down the wrong path.

Even our most natural bodily processes have been affected. Consider the medicalization of birth in this country. Whether they realize it or not, many American doctors are trained to "treat" pregnancy the same way they would treat any common illness. If you see pregnancy as a condition to be "remedied" using currently accepted protocols with varying levels of risk, this inevitably distorts your view of the entire process and how best to handle it. On the other hand, if you see birth as a natural process, you will take an entirely different approach.

As prominent ob-gyn, Michel Odent, has said, "We are completely lost. We have even forgotten to raise the most simple questions. What are the basic needs of women in labour?...The best thing to do is to go back to square one. The point of departure."[7] Once you've gone down the wrong path as a culture, it takes time to get everyone turned around moving in the right direction before you can make real progress forward. Most of that begins with education and changing false perceptions.

BECOMING PART OF THE SOLUTION

As with any cultural change, it begins with the individual. You can cultivate a growth mindset by asking the right questions. Remember, the quality of our questions informs the quality of our life.

Here are some great questions to ask about your health:

- Am I providing my body what it needs to be healthy? Is there any interference to its healing that I could remove?

- Do the medications I take actually make me healthier? Are there better, safer options?

- What role do I play in my own health? How have I developed my views on health? Where can I turn for sound advice on improving it?

- Do I trust the pills and potions marketed to me on TV more than the power that is beating my heart right now?

I recently had a conversation with a woman who was contemplating knee surgery. I offered findings from a study by *The New*

England Journal of Medicine indicating that surgery was no better than a placebo procedure (one where incisions are made but nothing is actually done to the joint).[8] Of course, she'd never heard this.

The woman's response spoke volumes about the larger problem: "Well, then where should I go to get it fixed?" This question reveals the common view of our bodies like broken-down cars and our entrenched bias toward the medical option, even when there's no proof it will work.

A better question would be, "What are my options?" In fact, there are many holistic, non-invasive, non-pharmaceutical approaches to try for knee pain. They might solve the problem, they might not—but if risky drugs and surgery have not been proven effective, why would you consider those first (or at all)?

In general, drug benefits are wildly overstated. Meanwhile, there are many effective and affordable things anyone can do to improve their health and aid the body's ability to heal itself, instead of chasing quick, expensive treatments with limited benefits and numerous side effects.

Whether a surgery or treatment is covered by insurance should not be the deciding factor. If it can't be proven significantly more effective than a placebo, it has no positive value. As I've shown, there is instead a high cost, both financially and in potential damage done to your body—not to mention the wasted time, stress, and energy spent on multiple doctor visits, tests, and treatments.

To truly improve health and lower costs, we have to engage and educate ourselves and those around us, as well as provide the resources, incentives, and opportunities proven to affect outcomes. A volleyball court and yoga studio will not lead to lasting change. Knowledge and follow-through will.

In 1902, Thomas Edison predicted that "the doctor of the future will give no medicine, but will instruct his patient in the care of the human frame, in diet, and in the cause and prevention of disease." As with so many other things, Edison was prescient in saying this, but his "future" is now upon us.

In the following chapters, I will lay out a vision for the health-care of the future—one that takes us back to the basics. But this is more than a case of the pendulum swinging the other direction, it is building on experience and learning from mistakes to chart a better course for generations to come.

CHAPTER TWO

Achieving Health through Cooperation

"Non-cooperation with evil is as much a duty as is cooperation with good." — Mahatma Gandhi

The human body is one of the most powerful examples of cooperation you can find. Its daily operations are more intricate and incredible than any machine or institution designed by man.

Have you ever wondered how you keep breathing when you fall asleep? Why your body even needs sleep? How a cut on your finger heals? It's estimated that of the 10 million bits of information our brains process each second, our consciousness can only handle about fifty of these bits.[9] Fifty!

This puts into perspective just how powerful our bodies are. We should literally be in awe of them. It also illustrates how unlikely it is that we can outsmart or manipulate the body to better health. Instead, let's focus on cooperation—which means not messing them up! It's a classic case of mistakenly trying to fix something that doesn't need fixing. The best health solution is not found down the path of "figuring out the human body," but by honoring the incredible inborn wisdom it contains.

The best way to take care of any living organism is to simply provide it what it needs. Erroneously however, we tend to do the opposite. Often, we expose the body to things it doesn't need to live or thrive (excessive sugar, large amounts of alcohol, smoking, exposure to chemicals, sedentary lifestyle, etc.) and then wonder why we get sick. If you poured toxic chemicals over a plant, would you be surprised when it started to wilt?

TAKING CARE OF WHAT WE'VE BEEN GIVEN

The power in this understanding is that now you have the proper perspective on where to spend most of your time and energy for your health and reversal of disease. Simply give your body what it needs to be healthy. The good news is that 99.9 percent of the hard work has already been done for you. It's like someone has dropped a Ferrari off in your driveway. It's already beautifully built. You wouldn't fill the gas tank with sugar and blame the car for not working right. All you need to do is take care of it.

However, there is one critical difference between cars and humans—*life*. It's beyond us to know exactly how it all works, but we cannot deny it exists. It's that spark, that power, that "electricity" that runs through our bodies. I personally know of no other way to explain it other than as a miracle of God.

This life, this power in your body, has healing capabilities (unlike the gas-fueled motor of a car). A car can't heal or fix itself. Maybe that's why we often take better care of our cars than our bodies.

We take our health for granted. We assume our bodies will keep putting up with the abuse we put them through. And for the most part, they do.

The body actually does an incredible job of keeping us as healthy as possible. However, when our bodies finally do show signs of abuse, *then* we treat them like cars and take them to the shop to get "fixed." We've got it backward.

Consider what many American's do to their bodies each day: eat fast food and ultra-processed food, slam a six-pack, have a few smokes, and live on coffee and soda in between (but don't forget your vitamins!). Then we wonder why we're sick, tired, or have high blood pressure! At this rate, it's only through the self-healing qualities of the body that we're still alive—a car would have died a long time ago.

What I find even more incredible—and promising—is when a symptom does show up (diabetes, high cholesterol, etc.), if you begin to properly care for your body, amazing things happen. The body will often completely heal and recover. What the body does when it has what it needs is pretty miraculous!

This healing power isn't a license for unhealthy living—our lifestyle eventually takes a toll. Remember being a kid? Living on candy bars, McDonald's, and sodas, but still feeling well enough to play all day? As adults, we often don't associate those lifestyle habits with the disease because we've been doing them so long we don't realize they're related.

Here's how this mentality plays out. It's been shown that each cigarette can take as much as 14 minutes off your life.[10] We don't tend to take this seriously because we don't see those immediate effects, but if you actually dropped dead for several minutes after every cigarette, you may seriously consider not having another one. Instead, the body's inborn detox systems will desperately try to help handle and remove the toxins behind the scenes, and smokers keep puffing away.

It's incredible that millions of people smoke for decades without getting cancer. Or that a person can be a lifelong alcoholic without experiencing liver failure. What's more, if alcoholics and smokers were to kick their habits, in most cases the body could heal and recover as if they never had abused these substances!

Now before you conclude that this means there's no harm in living recklessly for a while, think again. Just because you're not actively expressing disease or symptoms does not mean you're healthy. If I smoked three packs a day and lived on Snickers bars and Mountain Dew but had no symptoms of illness, should I be considered healthy? Of course not! You're not healthy just because you don't have heart disease or a cancer diagnosis—yet. Look at your lifestyle. You are either building health, or building disease.

Our "Ferraris" are designed to run for 300,000 miles yet we're wearing them out at 50,000—then saying we got a lemon. We must appreciate the role we play in our health (and disease) to better understand the potential that exists.

You might ask whether this applies to most diseases and health concerns, or just a handful of the more obvious and common cause-and-effect cases. I can't state it more emphatically—your body is designed to heal itself. Period. As a matter of fact, this may be the most powerful information in this book for some readers. So before we move on, let's get our foundation solid.

THE COOPERATIVE HEALTH MODEL

Your body is made up of trillions of cells. These cells comprise your organs and glands, which together make systems, which make—you. When your body is not functioning or healing optimally, it's due to decreased levels of cooperation. Something is out of sync. This is where many people begin to get off track, or misled.

Instead of ignoring the issue or popping a pill that masks what's really going on, the best solution would be to do things that enhance cooperation, rather than add interference.

Fostering cooperation takes time and effort (try mediating between two children fighting over a toy), but it's the right thing to do. Taking the time to cultivate cooperation in the body takes time and effort too, but it's the correct approach. It may *seem* easier to live carelessly than to make healthy choices, but there's nothing easy about suffering, disease, and pain.

It's crucial that we partner with our bodies in providing what they need. Partnership is very similar to cooperation. Both concepts embody the same principles: parts and pieces working together for a common goal. Imagine a machine with 200 gears designed to work together, but no power or electricity to move them. Not much would happen. But if we connect a motor to the gears, we have a system that could accomplish significant tasks.

Similarly, a body with all the parts and pieces is just a dead body, but when it has the "spark of life," everything changes! It's the God-given power that controls and organizes your body. It's like having a perfect CEO on the job at all times, that never sleeps, never makes mistakes, and works for free. However, the CEO can only work with what's provided, and that's up to you.

This is where being a good partner comes in. As we'll see, part of this means being an advocate for your body and seeking out the right external partners and resources. Health and wellness is no different on a personal level than an organizational level. You can apply the same principles of cooperation and partnership. Finding a core group of people that can encourage you helps to add oil to the gears of cooperation.

With that in mind, let's look at three key areas of the cooperative wellness model:

- NUTRITION
  There is a nutritional aspect to health and disease. It is well worth your time to have a core understanding of nutrition and the needs of your body. Get to know the local farmers' markets, the healthy restaurants, the co-ops or grocery stores where you can get good, healthy food. It is also a great idea to find some trusted resources for nutritional advice. Avoid fad diets and stick to the basics.

- FITNESS
  Motion is life! There are countless benefits to regular physical activity. This could be another book in itself, but finding a way to move your body and break a sweat on a regular basis is irreplaceable.

- HEALTHCARE PROVIDER
  It's important to have a healthcare provider that is aligned with your beliefs as it relates to health. I have countless stories of people I've worked with that wanted non-drug, natural solutions to get to the cause of their problem, yet found themselves in a medical system that prescribed dangerous drugs for almost every condition. It cannot be overstated how important this is. If you want incredible health, find a doctor or healthcare expert that actually focuses on *health* and offers natural solutions that get to the cause.

BUT IT'S TOO EXPENSIVE

Unfortunately, we often make health decisions based on economics. Remember though, one of the core principles of the cooperative health model is that it *all works together* for the greater good—this includes economics. You'll not only find this to be true on a personal level, but also in a corporate setting—integrating cooperative solutions can be beneficial in countless ways, including financially.

Ultimately, the only way we are going to lower the cost of providing medical care and improving our health – individually and collectively – is to be well enough to use less medical care.

A significant portion of lowering medical usage is proper self-care, prevention, wellness, and lifestyle. However, many of us still unnecessarily participate in the medical system more than we are aware of. We don't realize we're on the slippery slope of medical care.

Back pain, for instance, is one of the most common reasons for medical care. It affects millions of people each year, causing them to miss work and significantly limits their activity and lifestyle. The medical spending associated with back pain can be tremendous—expensive tests, expensive treatments, and often dangerous procedures.

Let's examine the typical medical approach. First, you "throw your back out." You try to tough it out for a few days but it's not improving, so you begin to take a few anti-inflammatory drugs (medical approach) and this seems to "help" (masking the pain). You feel better, so you begin to do the activities you were doing before. A week later, the pain returns. You pop a few pills, but they don't seem to help anymore. You finally go to the doctor—they suggest an x-ray. It shows some mild degeneration. They suggest an MRI. You get it. They tell you that you have a bulging disc. They recommend therapy and prescription pain pills. The therapy seems to help a little, but does not last. Then they say, "Well, I guess you need surgery." So you have a discectomy, attempt to recover, never really feel like yourself again, have chronic low back pain, and are now part of the statistic showing that, of the more than 500,000 disc surgeries performed annually, as many as 90 percent are unnecessary and ineffective.[11]

The scenario I just described has been shown to cost as much as $100,000 in total medical spending. Add this to the pile of nationwide medical costs, disability, work loss, and other indirect costs attributed to back pain, and you're looking at a staggering $100–200 billon annually.[11] This is a horrible return on investment in terms of both health and financial outcomes. There has to be a better way!

Now, let's take a look at the cooperative model. First, it starts by understanding that the body is intelligent. The pain you are experiencing is trying to warn you, not hurt you. It's not comfortable, but masking it with medications is rarely an intelligent decision, any more than covering up the check engine light or taking batteries out of the smoke alarm to keep it quiet. So how do we get to the cause of the problem? It's important to remember the body is already doing all it can to heal the problem. We want to find ways to support or cooperate with the healing your body is already doing. With that in mind, we could try some ice, gentle stretching, and natural support for inflammation (omega-3, vitamin D, bromelain) for a few days (most acute injuries will resolve on their own in three to seven days). If it does not show improvement in a few days, you may seek a natural, conservative healthcare provider—chiropractic adjustments are shown to be the most effective treatment for this type of back pain—better than drugs or acupuncture.[12] They may take x-rays, attempting to discover the underlying cause. They may provide conservative, natural care (adjustments, spinal rehabilitation, etc.).

This is generally done for a few hundred dollars, not thousands. In most cases, taking these steps will resolve the problem and is a better approach than the medical model. It follows the logical progression of cooperative healthcare—from least invasive to most invasive, as shown below.

PREVENTION → NATURAL → CONSERVATIVE → DRUGS → SURGERY

A large majority of many health problems can be avoided completely by engaging in preventative and proactive healthcare. For example, regular spinal adjustments offer countless benefits to overall health, including reducing or eliminating spinal decay and degeneration. I strongly encourage you to not simply use natural vitalistic healthcare to regain health—it's even more powerful to *maintain* health.

I think most people would agree with the idea of taking the least invasive approach first—they just don't know how to engage in the cooperative model. They go to the doctor and find themselves on the slippery slope of the medical model, and then believe they did "everything they could." They may have exhausted their options in the medical model, but let me assure you, there is far more to health and healing than drugs and surgery.

The medical model is incredibly expensive, often danger-ous, and not as effective as you are led to believe. Sadly, I could provide countless examples of the ineffectiveness of the medical model that we blindly follow because "the doctor said so" or "it's covered by insurance." We shouldn't be afraid to ask ques-tions. Does this work? Does it get to the cause? Are there other, safer options?

One reason this is so important for me to convey to others is because I wish I'd have asked those questions in my early years.

MY STORY

I grew up in the Midwest, South Dakota to be specific. We were a good, hardworking, middle-class family—the typical family in most respects. We ate the typical American diet, took the typical drugs when we were sick, went to medical clinics and hospitals, followed doctor's orders, etc. That's what you do, right? I never questioned it. It was my normal.

When I was around 10 years old, I was introduced to a sport that would change the direction of my life. A friend of my dad's was the local boxing coach. One day, as I was wrestling around with my dad, he asked if I would like to try boxing. I said yes, of course! Wouldn't any boy love to be able to beat people up and get trophies instead of getting in trouble?

I fell in love with the sport and enjoyed significant success over the years. I started boxing in the 85-pound weight class and worked my way to becoming one of the top-ranked light heavyweights in the United States. My dream was to make it to the 1996 Olympics.

I began attending camps during my late teen years at the Olympic training center and was working with past and future

Olympians, when all of the sudden I "got sick." My digestive system started to shut down. I felt terrible. Doctors ran scans and tests, then sat me down to tell me that I had precancerous lesions throughout my digestive system, and my only solution was medication.

I was scared. I didn't ask questions. I didn't think I had any other options. So I took the medications. This shut my digestive system down even further and I gained more than 70 pounds. My Olympic hopes were destroyed and I suffered down this route for three more years.

As I tell my story, I feel a flood of emotions. But something good came out of all of this. I was referred to a doctor who focused on health rather than disease. A doctor who, for the first time in my life, sat me down and explained how the body heals and functions. He explained that my body is designed to heal, and if it's not doing that, there must be a cause.

We began the process of finding the interference. In my case, there were two significant issues. Number one, the nerves that controlled my digestive system were interfered with. Much like the wire you plug into the wall to power your computer, if the power (nerves) are interfered with, the computer will not function properly. No drug can fix this. Number two, I needed to make some changes to my nutrition that were more aligned with how my body is designed. With God as my witness, after one week I was able to completely get off the medications I had been on for more than three years, I lost 67 pounds in four months, and my body returned to normal.

This was not only a life-saving, but a life-changing experience. It changed how I saw health, healthcare, and my body's ability to heal. I began to ask different questions such as, how did my body heal and function normally for so long? How did my body forget how to properly digest food? Why was the suggested solution for my symptoms to take two dangerous (in fact, life-threatening) medications for the rest of my life? It did not add up to me.

> It was later discovered that one of the drugs I'd been given killed 33,000 people a year.[13] Had I continued taking it, I may not be alive to tell you this story, or to kiss my wife and kids.

You may not be surprised to learn that this experience was part of what put me on the path of natural healthcare and ignited my passion for proposing a cooperative healthcare model.

For the past fifteen years, my family and I have rarely been to a medical doctor or hospital. It's simply not part of our lives. By choice, we participate in a different model of healthcare. There are zero medications in my home. My "medicine cabinet" is empty. I do not own a thermometer, cough syrup, or even Alka-Seltzer. Nothing. Following the vitalistic, cooperative healthcare model has left us with little need or use for the medical model. To some, this may seem extreme or even radical. I suggest it should be the norm.

Now let me be clear, my family occasionally "gets sick," but we heal up quickly, without the use of medical intervention. We have had minor (and a few major) health issues over the years, but we were able to get to the cause and find solutions naturally, cooperatively.

You can have the same experience. Yes, as a natural healthcare provider, my education has significantly helped me understand this model and how to use it, but I have taught thousands to do the same. I highly suggest you find a natural wellness practitioner to be your primary doctor that can come alongside you in this way.

I have one other significant advantage. I have watched tens of thousands of people recover and heal outside of the traditional medical model. I witness "miracles" daily. I have seen chronic disease disappear. I have seen people move from fear to hope. I have worked with other doctors around the world and witnessed their patients' recoveries as well.

> Every time I see health restored, it strengthens my understanding and faith in a vitalistic health model.

I have moved beyond merely suggesting this model as an "alternative" and into the reality that this is simply the best practice to care for the body we have been given. A holistic, cooperative, vitalistic approach should be our primary healthcare model, not a last resort. We must move past seeing healthcare as a mechanic shop for broken cars and on to a new view of healthcare as partnering with our bodies to provide what they need.

Perhaps some of you have possibly written me off as overzealous, crazy, or a quack. (Thank you for continuing to read anyway. I assure you, I have been called worse.) But I am obligated to share and speak out on behalf of the sick and suffering—and those yet to be. I was once unaware that this approach even existed until someone taught me about true health and healing. It changed everything for me. And it can do the same for you.

LIGHTENING THE LOAD

My dad had a dog named Pepper. He loved Pepper very much, but really didn't know much about taking care of dogs. If my dad liked a certain food, he figured it was probably good for the dog too.

One day, Dad found cans of beef stew on sale and thought it would be great for Pepper. A couple of weeks later, the dog began to behave differently. He was having accidents, couldn't get comfortable, and just overall seemed sick. My dad took Pepper to the veterinarian and the first question the vet asked was, "What are you feeding him?"

Doesn't it seem like such an obvious question? He didn't give him three different drugs for each symptom. The problem was caused by what the dog was eating, therefore the only intelligent cure would be to correct his diet. So my dad did, and guess what—Pepper healed up.

Why is it so hard for us to apply the same wisdom to human healthcare? I think it's a combination of things. For many years, we were told it didn't really matter what we ate, and most of the nutrition advice revolved around obesity. Today, we are becoming acutely aware of the direct connection between food and disease. The food you eat becomes your body. It's that simple. And that amazing.

The other influence is more cultural. More and more, people do not want to take responsibility for their lives. Even suggesting the idea that our lifestyle decisions are making us sick can rub some people the wrong way. But we are life-styling ourselves to death. We need to reframe disease and understand how lifestyles contribute.

Smoking is a classic example. We understand you won't get lung cancer from smoking a single cigarette, but rather cancer develops over time as a person continues to be exposed to the toxic chemicals.

At some point, the body cannot keep up or recover, and cancer (abnormal cell growth) develops in response to the carcinogens.

It's like carrying rocks in your backpack. I first heard this concept from Dr. James Chestnut, a researcher on health and wellness.[14] It's a simple metaphor of a complicated concept—allostasis.

Allostasis refers to the burden or stress load that our bodies are under. The more stress (all types) we have, the higher our allostaic load, the more likely we are to suffer from disease or have health-related problems. It's the old straw that breaks the camel's back.

This powerful metaphor dramatically simplifies the conversations we need to have regarding our health. Instead of treating the symptoms caused by carrying the heavy backpack, we attempt to get to the cause of the problem by removing rocks from the backpack so the body can heal (cooperate) better.

Almost all stress can be broken down into three simple categories—physical, chemical, and emotional. Rocks all go into the same backpack. The more stress in any or all of these areas, the more potential for disease we will have. However, the opposite is also true, improving even one of these areas often helps you feel and heal better overall. For example, eating better can improve your mood and your weight. Exercising can improve both your emotional and physical health, because they're directly related. This is good news, and reinforces the power of a holistic model of care.

What if we had a health program that focused on working *with* the body, instead of working against it? An approach that begins with the premise that the body is smart and designed to heal? An understanding that our best shot at health doesn't come by doing more but by interfering less? What if the prevailing view of healthcare focused on lightening our load?

A healthcare model like this would be nothing short of a revolution on par with the civil rights movement. Martin Luther King Jr. shared his vision for civil rights in the famous "I Have a Dream" speech. He envisioned a place where people are not judged by the color of their skin, but the content of their character. People far too often take things at face value and stop short of the truth that lies within.

Our nation needs to be swept up by another such dream that stems from truth rather than assumption. A dream of a healthcare model built on cooperation, not manipulation. A model that's based on achieving wellness, not focused on the dollar bill. A model that does not exclude natural healthcare (or at best sidetrack it as alternative option that comes with an additional cost), but places it at the front of the treatment progression.

I have a dream for a healthcare model that understands this: The best doctor in the world lives inside you. Continuing to rely on prescription medication may seem scientific, but is really the genie-in-a-bottle approach—rather than wishing for a quick (superficial) "fix," let's work together toward the dream of achieving true wellness.

INFLUENCE WORKS

If someone had predicted 50 years ago that we would be taking medications for everything from thicker eyelashes to toenail fungus, that nearly 60 percent of American adults[15] and 25 percent of our kids[16] would be taking prescription drugs, few would have believed it. But that's exactly where we sit.

How did this occur right under our noses?

In 2013, Big Pharma, the largest lobbying group in the U.S., spent $226 million and employed an army of 1,500 lobbyists on Capitol Hill, spending $422,000 per congressman.[17] Do you think this influences laws, access, marketing, rules, and insurance? You'd better believe it.

One FDA study found that nearly 50 percent of patients who had recently seen a doctor and remembered seeing a prescription drug ad had inquired about the drug—in more than half of those cases, it was for a condition they'd never asked about before. About 75 percent of doctors said the ads cause patients to think a drug works better than it does, 60 percent believed patients did not understand the risks, and 20 percent felt somewhat pressured to prescribe the specific brand name when asked to do so.[18]

If this is how adults are affected, imaging the impact on our children as they grow up in the age of ever-increasing drug advertising. Kids are led to believe that "medicine" equals "healthy" through drug-sponsored vehicles like "educational" comic books (designed to be handed out in classrooms) and even smartphone apps. This doesn't begin to cover the more subtle effects of what kids hear and see on TV. One study found that children viewed TV ads for erectile dysfunction an estimated 30 billion times between 2006 and 2010.[19]

Advertising works — that's why billions are spent each year on drug campaigns. This should deeply concern us. If we're led to believe drugs are healthy, it follows that we feel like we're doing the right thing by taking them.

We think we're doing the right thing by medicating our symptoms. We think we're doing the right thing by taking cholesterol drugs and blood pressure medication and acid reflux pills and depression meds.

But we're wrong.

A NEW DOSE – REALITY

If drugs work so well, we should be healthier than ever. It's simply not true. As a matter of fact, the opposite is true. Study after study is showing that, collectively, our nation's health is on the decline. The 2015 Annual Report by America's Health Rankings found that the U.S. ranks at or near the bottom among high-income countries on nearly all indicators of mortality, survival, and life expectancy.[20]

I firmly believe, if people understood the ineffectiveness of medications to truly heal (not to mention the countless side effects) and grasped the impact of their lifestyle choices on the body's ability to heal, there would be a revolution based on these revelations alone.

One of my heroes, William Wilberforce, led the abolition of slavery and slave trade in Europe. He took people into the gallows of slave trade ships. He made them see, taste, and smell the reality of slavery. He made them face the horror of what was going on beneath the surface. He forced them to question: Was slavery really right?

The same thing must continue to be done as it relates to today's healthcare model. Although these conversations can be uncomfortable, in order to have meaningful change in healthcare, we must deal with the realities. We need to look beyond the shiny marble hospital floors and the attractive prescription drug reps to see the underbelly of the industrial medical complex. It's not pretty.

One of the most disturbing things I've noticed is that people feel like they "have to do something" as it relates to healthcare. We are often made to feel like we are stupid or negligent if we don't "follow doctor's orders," even though many times, doctor's orders are nothing more than Big Pharma and insurance companies' directives. This is beyond a dangerous model; it's outright criminal, and it's certainly not healthcare. What if doctors were paid for keeping you off drugs instead of on them?

If you and I want healthcare to be better, more affordable, easier, and safer, we need to make different decisions.

Our nation makes up only 5 percent of the world's population, yet we consume 80 percent of the world's prescription painkillers.[21] About three out of every five American adults take some sort of prescription drug.[15]

I will make a bold assertion—we have been brainwashed. We have been manipulated. There have been billions of dollars spent every year for the last 20-plus years, convincing us that drug prescriptions are the solution to our ills! We have swallowed this pill (pun intended).

What if, instead of consuming the most drugs, our nation began consuming the most vegetables? What if, instead of getting little-to-no regular exercise, we became active? Do you think we would be healthier? You bet! And yet, this common sense seems quickly discarded when we're sick. It's time to move from holistic healthcare being a good idea, to being the accepted primary model of care.

Instead of having ambulances ready at the bottom of a cliff, it makes more sense to put up warning signs, offer driving classes, and install guardrails. The same is true of healthcare—let's focus on wellness and prevention. The battle cry is simple: We need to take responsibility for our own health and actions. The best medical approach is staying well. In my opinion, the only safe drug is none. (Yes, there's a time and a place for medical care, and we'll touch on this a bit later, but it's significantly—significantly—less than most of us realize.)

We sit at a unique time in history. We're living through a health-care revolution. It's up to us, as individuals, as organizations, to determine what the outcome will be.

Will we continue to close our eyes tight, open our mouths wide, and take their pills as directed? Or will we engage in and demand a holistic, vitalistic, cooperative model of care? It seems like an easy choice to me. The challenge is turning the tide, so let's take a closer look at how that can happen.

CHAPTER THREE

Are You Cooperating?

"Nature needs no help...just no interference." — B.J. Palmer

Consider this: All of the scientists in the entire world, through the history of time, have never created one single living cell from scratch. I will go so far as to say they never will.

The spark of life is a mystery. It's bigger than us. We do not create life, that's not our job—our job is to take care of it. Although we often think of the body as a machine (as in our car analogy), in reality it is much more complex. A more accurate comparison would be an ecosystem, or perhaps a garden.

THE GIFT OF GRACE

If our bodies were not so incredible at healing, we would all be dead by now. Imagine if every poor health decision you have made was still with you. Have you ever thought about the incredible amount of resilience your body has? If you scratch or dent your car door, the damage is still going to be there in the morning. If you hurt your body, whether by accident or lifestyle choices, there is a really good chance (if given what it needs) that it will heal and recover. It's kind of like a self-healing car. Wouldn't that be great—imagine the money you could save!

You may falsely believe that you're going to have to live perfectly to be healthy. This is simply not the case. Of course, the closer you align your lifestyle choices with the needs of your body, the better you will function. This is not false hope or wishful thinking. If we were actually aware of how much healing our bodies do on a daily basis just to keep us functioning, we would be in awe. The answer always has been, and always will be, to work with your body.

THE AHA MOMENT

I remember the first time I walked into the cadaver lab while I was studying for my doctorate. I was not looking forward to it. I know this may sound odd coming from a doctor who's writing a book about the healing power within us, but it's the truth. I can still smell the formaldehyde and see the lifeless cadavers lying on stainless steel tables. These were people who had generously donated their bodies to science. They varied in age and cause of death. We spent the next year working through the process of dissecting a human body. It was an experience that changed my life.

When we had finally removed the outer layers of skin, fat, and muscle, we began to get to the organs—that's when it hit me. The incredibly intricate design, the interrelatedness, the coordination and cooperation of the human body, is beyond comprehension. The divine design was unquestionable to me at this moment. I literally have goose bumps as I write this. I realized right then and there that, as a doctor, I was unable to heal people, but what I could do was teach them about the incredible design and healing power within them. I also realized that our absolute best chance at health and healing comes from working with the healing power within us, rather than attempting to manipulate the body with drugs and surgery. This was my aha moment. The moment I understood that the power of a pill compared to the power in a living human being is like comparing a grain of sand to all the beaches of the world. And that still gives too much credit to the grain of sand.

> When you look inside a body and see the intimacy and intricacy of the design, it literally takes your breath away. You realize that the trillions of things that need to happen every second for a body to exist are way beyond our understanding, and always will be.

That moment, standing over the table, looking at God's divine design, instantly put into perspective the role each of us plays in health.

That role is to honor, to support, to be good stewards, to cooperate with our bodies. The future of healthcare is not growing organs in test tubes to replace organs we damaged by our destructive lifestyles. The future of healthcare is honoring the bodies we have. The body that was designed specifically for each of us. By properly caring for our bodies, we significantly reduce the need for medical intervention and thereby lower healthcare costs. We also enjoy the benefits of improved health and wellness along the way! There is no down side. We will have less disease, better health, less medical spending, better function, less fear of sickness. It's how healthcare should be, and it *is* possible.

You may not have the opportunity to look inside a human body, but I hope this book helps you have your aha moment. One of the definitions of doctor is "teacher"—I could not agree more. As we navigate this journey together, I pray that I am living up to that definition. I pray that you have a moment where you put the book down for a few seconds because you are in awe, overwhelmed by this deep truth of health and healing—that the blinders are ripped from your eyes and you are freed from any medical marketing deception. I hope you are able to see the gift we've been given, and the role we play in caring for it.

When that happens, it's like a switch flips. You see the world differently. You begin to see that taking medications in an attempt to be healthier doesn't make sense (except maybe as a last resort, in extreme circumstances), and we begin to understand our role in removing interference.

When your eyes are opened to the truth, healthcare becomes something you do, not a building, insurance card, or a pill bottle. You begin to view healthcare as the daily decisions you make to get well and stay well.

So let me ask you, do you have more faith in a pill than you do in the power that's causing your heart to beat right now? What would it take for you to step outside of the traditional medical model? Working with patients over the years, I've been surprised by how strongly some people would cling to ineffective, expensive, and dangerous medical models of care, instead of a more natural approach. I've often asked people what it would take to change their minds and found that most of them simply did not know there were valid, evidence-based alternatives.

Sometimes what you don't know, *can* hurt you.

When the Vioxx prescription drug disaster was uncovered, there was admitted fraud and deception involved. It's estimated that more than 160,000 were injured and 38,000 people lost their lives in the name of profit.[22] In my mind, this was nothing short of murder. How else do you describe the action of delivering a non-life-saving drug to more than 25 million people, while knowing it was dangerous?

Many people I've talked to are frustrated with the endless marketing and massive drive for profits, yet still sign on for dangerous medications, tests, or surgeries. Maybe it's because they don't know where else to turn. Let's look at some basic changes you can make to begin to create different results.

THE BASICS

Does your current healthcare approach align with the cooperative model? Do you see your body as an incredible, self-healing, intricate, powerful, amazing, cooperating organism that is trying its best to heal and function and do all it can with what it's being given?

Or do you more often find yourself frustrated and upset with your body or health? Do you find yourself blaming your body? Do you look in the mirror or your medicine cabinet and wonder, "How did I get here?" If this describes you, I am so grateful you are reading this book. Once you begin to search for solutions from the perspective of "How can I cooperate with my body?" everything changes.

Imagine this patient/doctor conversation:

DOCTOR: You have diabetes.

PATIENT: Why?

DOCTOR: Because you have high blood sugar.

PATIENT: Why?

DOCTOR: Because you have diabetes!

Do you see the flawed thinking? This reveals the circular reasoning that often prevents us from getting to the cause of the problem. It also prevents us from taking ownership of the problem or concern.

The following simple analogy can help you think through most health challenges:

- THE PROBLEM
  If I have a rock in my shoe and it's causing me pain and discomfort, what options do I have to relieve it? What action is most likely to get to the cause of the problem?

- OPTION #1
  What if I took some pain pills or used chemicals to mask the pain? Would the problem still be there? Yes. Even though I wouldn't feel it as much, or at all; the rock is still there, potentially causing further damage.

- OPTION #2
  What if I took off my shoe and massaged my foot for a while? Would that feel good? Yes! When I put the shoe back on (with the rock still inside), what will happen? The pain returns.

- OPTION #3
  What if I just cut off the foot? The pain from the rock would be gone, but now I only have one foot left.

- OPTION #4
  Take the rock out of the shoe.

Although this is such an obvious example, it explains the majority of the health solutions we need. There is no disease that exists because of a lack of medication or chemicals. Thus, the solution by definition will never be drugs. Let's pause here for a second to let this sink in. Do drugs have effects? Yes. Can they alter physiology or mask symptoms or pain? Yes. Do they get to the cause of the problem? No.

To put this in perspective, let's look at it outside the realm of prescription drugs. What if I was very tired but had a lot of work to do, so I decided to do some cocaine as a pick-me-up?. Or let's say I'm stressed out, so I decided to have a bottle of whiskey for dinner. Would I possibly feel less stress for a few hours? Maybe. But did I address the stress? No. The cause of the problem was not a cocaine or whiskey deficiency!

We can save a lot of time, money, and energy when we understand the basic needs of a human body. Remember our plant analogy? If you provide for its basic needs, chances are, the plant is going to live a healthy life. If you take any of those basic needs away for too long, the overall health of the plant will suffer and disease will start to show up. The human body is similar in that it has basic needs. When these needs are met, the body will be as healthy as possible and any diseases related directly or indirectly to lifestyle will be resolved or prevented.

Let's review the basic needs of human physiology:

- NUTRITION
  Garbage in, garbage out. What you eat matters.

- MOVEMENT
  Life is motion. Less motion, less life. No motion, death.

- EMOTIONAL HEALTH OR PURPOSE
  Our state of mind is directly related to our state of health.

When these basic needs are met, we thrive. When the needs are not met for an extended period of time, our health is compromised—diseases and conditions may begin to appear. However, the good news is that when you provide the body with its basics needs again, it can often heal, much like the wilted brown leaves of a plant coming back to life.

Oftentimes, our lack of understanding and appreciation about the healing power of the body leads us down an ineffective medical path. Improving blood pressure, digestion issues, high cholesterol, blood sugar, etc. (symptoms of lifestyle) may take some time, but these health issues can very often be helped or resolved. Most people that struggle with common health problems today have simply never had a person educate them and walk them through the process of getting to the root of the problem. They didn't even know it was possible.

ARE THERE EXCEPTIONS?

"But what about...?" This seems to be the question I hear so many times regarding health challenges and the typical medical approach. This is also the justification we use (or is used against us) to push us into medical tests and procedures.

Birth usually is at the top of the list of "exceptions" people worry about addressing outside of the traditional model. First of all, birth is not a disease—it's a natural process. The woman's body is designed to grow and deliver a baby. That's a fact proven billions of times over. The entire approach to supporting a birth should operate out of this premise. Unfortunately, almost the opposite is true and birth is treated like a disease. There is significant evidence to show how poorly the U.S. is medically managing birth.[23] It's a tragic example of how the ego- and profit-driven medical model has not improved a natural process, but rather hurt it.

"But what about a birth emergency?"

Yes, there are many, many, *many* things we do on a daily basis that can cause an emergency. Thousands of people choke to death every year, but we don't require people to eat all their meals in a hospital. Beyond this mistaken, fear-based rationale, statistics show that there is something amiss with our approach.

C-sections are through the roof (more than 33 percent), medical interventions are at an all-time high, associated costs are out of control — and still, U.S. infant and maternal mortality rates are some of the worst in the industrialized world.[23]

All this money spent, all the time and energy invested in intervention and worry—and we're not making things better, but actually making them worse. It doesn't add up. There are dozens of countries that have much better birth outcomes than we do, for a fraction of the cost. Our approach sets off a domino effect of more problems such as decreased breastfeeding, increased long-term risks for mom and baby, and the medical merry-go-round continues.

Whether we're talking birth or taking a trip to the ER for aches and pains, actual emergencies are few and far between. One study showed that 71 percent of emergency department visits are unnecessary, with an average cost of $1,316.[24] This illustrates not only how broken our system is, but also how fear can cloud our thinking.

The reality is that even with all of our visits to doctor's offices and hospitals, all of our tests, all of our drugs—as a nation, we're actually getting sicker.

Studies reveal:

- Many screening tests can do more harm than good, and certainly are not 100 percent accurate (mammograms, prostate, etc.).[25]

- Annual physicals at $10 billion a year have shown to be a waste of money (but good profit).[26]

- Medications are toxic chemicals and merely treat symptoms instead of getting to the cause. Medications do not make a person healthier, but can cause serious adverse reactions, including death.[27]

- Each year, 7.5 million unnecessary medical and surgical procedures are performed.[27]

We must wake up. We must see the medical model for what it is—an expensive, chemical, profit-driven approach with limited results and a very poor track record of improving health. Each of us must take responsibility for our own health. We must search out solutions that work with the body and get to the cause of the problem.

After people begin learning about this holistic approach, a common question I hear is, "Should I continue to see my MD?" This is a decision each of us needs to make for ourselves, but here are some good questions to consider:

- Are you interested in taking medications or having surgery for what they may diagnose you with?

- Will having a diagnosis (naming the problem) really help?

- Can you feel confident that the diagnosis will be correct?

- Do you understand that going to see a doctor and doing what they recommend is *your* choice? There is no law that requires you to seek medical attention, nor to follow "doctor's orders."

- Why do you want to go? Are you scared? Looking for reassurance?

For a growing number of people, seeing a medical doctor is not their approach to health. They don't actually care what the name of the condition or disease is, and they don't want the drugs, tests, or surgery the doctors are going to suggest. Instead, they look at their lifestyles, get some advice from some natural healthcare providers, find ways to add health or remove interference, and give it some time.

However, there are still many people who have never attempted a cooperative model of healthcare. Every day, someone has a neck ache, gets an MRI, finds a bulging disc, and assumes the medical suggestions given are the best options. When drugs don't work and shots don't work, it's time to try surgery and hope for the best. This limited approach is having a serious impact on our ability to get and stay well.

Less-invasive methods aren't even on the radar. Perhaps they seem too simple. Or perhaps some people decide they take too much time and effort. It's like wanting to lose weight, eating one salad, jogging around the block, and then stepping on the scale to conclude that diet and exercise don't work.

But most of us know diet and exercise *do* work, and the same principle applies to a vitalistic model of healthcare. We often just don't give our bodies enough credit, and instead erroneously put our trust in medication instead.

Almost every condition or symptom has a non-drug solution. We often give medication the credit for healing, when in fact, the body healed in spite of the medications — not because of them.

It's important to ask the following questions before taking any medications:

- What are the effects of this drug? It may make me feel better, but will I heal better?
- What are the side effects?
- What might be the long-term effects?
- Does this medication get to the cause of my problem?
- What costs are involved?
- What could I do instead?

ARE NATURAL "REMEDIES" BETTER THAN DRUGS?

Let's take a moment to discuss natural treatments. Once people understand that most medications are simply a Band-Aid or masking the problem, they instead look to treat the problem using natural approaches. While this is often safer, due to the reduction of toxic effects from drugs, you may still wind up masking or manipulating instead of cooperating with the body.

For example, there are natural substances you can take in an effort to lower cholesterol—red yeast rice is one of them. However, the substances in red yeast rice react much the same way statin drugs do (which are harmful to the liver) and you're still not getting to the cause of the problem.

Your body does not have a red yeast rice deficiency any more than it has a Lipitor deficiency.

Here are two questions to ask when considering natural solutions:

- Is this improving a deficiency (for example, low vitamin D)?

- Is this safely removing something that is interfering (detox, for example)?

Remember, the most natural approach of all (and the best approach in a vast majority of cases), is to provide your body what it needs and then leave matters to the greatest doctor of all. Where does such a doctor live?

How does the cut on your finger heal? How does the food you ate yesterday turn into new body parts tomorrow? The healing power inside us that is constantly at work and cooperating for our good is more powerful than anything else when it comes to health, healing, wellness, and prevention.

It bears repeating: The greatest doctor in the world lives inside of you!

Side note: There are certain health crises that may require more advanced interventions. That is not a discussion for this book. However, they are available and can be very powerful for short-term, crisis situations. They should not be part of a wellness or prevention approach to health over the long term.

CHAPTER FOUR

Cooperating Makes Cents (and Dollars)

"[Man] sacrifices his health in order to make money. Then he sacrifices money to recuperate his health." – Dalai Lama

Now that we've established a foundation for the cooperative approach, let's turn our attention to how this plays out financially. How does a holistic model of care save you or your company money? In the same way that oil changes and regular home maintenance allow you to get the best results from those investments, regular care of your body will dramatically reduce, or even prevent, health problems. This is not simply wishful thinking, it's a logical, well-established, scientifically supported fact.

Since a significant majority of today's health problems are diseases of lifestyle—the consequences of living against the natural design of the body—we hold the key that opens the door to healthy living. This, in turn, will reduce our medical burden both physically and economically. Once we take full responsibility for our health, we are no longer unlucky victims that merely manage, cope, and drift helplessly through the medical system. The cooperative approach fosters confidence—you can support your body's inborn ability to heal and get the best results for your health.

Does all of this sound too good to be true? Or even too simple? It should! Many of the greatest truths seem so simple once they're revealed.

As mentioned, the civil rights struggle is a fitting analogy to the current healthcare crisis. Not many years ago, the color of a person's skin played a large role in the perception of their value to humankind. Although we are still facing struggles around the globe in regard to racism and civil rights, significant progress has been made. The vision of civil rights was very simple: All people are created equal.

We sit at a similar place in healthcare. What holds us back is a mixed bag of misunderstanding and fear of change—many people are wired to stay in a perceived "comfort" zone, even if it's uncomfortable! We cannot simply sweep this under the rug or ignore the problems that the medicalization of society is causing. Healthcare is due for a revolution. The simple premise is that the body is designed to be healthy. The best healthcare model must support this.

DEVELOPING A LEAN MINDSET

The concept of creating efficiencies and dissolving bottlenecks is crucial. When it comes to healthcare and the amount of individual and corporate spending associated with it, we must evaluate it from a lean mindset.

Here's the question we should ask: How do we provide and participate in a brilliant healthcare model and spend less doing so? The simple answer is to use less medicine. With lean management principles, whenever you appear to be taking something away, people will often have an initial response to hold on tight. And so it is with healthcare. The (false) perception of many consumers is if we had cheaper drugs, tests, and insurance, we would all be healthier.

No one asks if this medical approach actually works. A cheaper broken model, is still broken. We must be willing to make a shift. Corporate America (the people who fund almost all healthcare through taxes and wages) has to be brave and smart enough to step up and say enough is enough. If you're the passionate sort, you might even quote the movie *Network:* "I'm as mad as hell, and I'm not going to take this anymore!"[28]

The medical-industrial complex and its pharmaceutical approach to health is shortsighted, incomplete, expensive, and greedy. Even the Mayo Clinic's former president and CEO, Dr. Denis Cortese, admitted there's a problem. "Trying to make tweaks to the current system is really doomed for failure," he said. "There really is no system of health care in this country now."[29]

Need I say more?

If I asked 100 random people whether they should take care of their health, I think almost every one of them would say yes.

> We all know we should take better care of ourselves, but at the same time, culture tells us to not worry about it—supersize it, take this pill, it's not your fault, it's genetic.

The media-driven, deep cultural beliefs that many people are brainwashed to accept as truth are instead lies that are on par with the comments made by influential people in the past regarding the color of a person's skin.

We can no longer deny the effects of this type of thinking. Ignorance is bliss, but it's also deadly. We must see our role in solving this both personal and corporate problem. There will never be a shortcut in caring for what the good Lord gave you. A face-lift may make you look younger, but it doesn't make you healthier.

Doing the right thing isn't always easy, but it's simple—and it's worth it. Fostering cooperation—whether we're talking civil rights or health—is worth it. We've seen the impact of the alternative course: a way of life that is unsustainable, expensive, ineffective, and deadly.

Instead, imagine a culture of people and businesses guided by an understanding of holistic, vitalistic principles, and given access to a conservative clinical model that operates from this paradigm. This would radically change the health and economics of this great nation.

As companies and individuals, we must be willing to explore new models that are outside of the industrial medical complex to allow for increased health and wellness. We must maintain the willingness to push the bounds of standard medical practice and take back healthcare. Remember, it's *your* health—and if you're an employer, you can also impact the health of your employees, which is crucial to your business.

Embracing the cooperative model is not such an intimidating leap when we remember that we did not create our bodies, but the God who did works for our good, always. Every time I consider this, it humbles me as a doctor and helps put in perspective where the focus needs to be in healthcare.

Regardless of your personal spiritual convictions, the understanding of our body's innate power to heal itself should be the backbone of our healthcare model.

COOPERATION IN A GROUP CONTEXT

Let's look at how the cooperative model works with groups of people. Philosophically and logically, I believe we could agree that a healthy workplace and healthy employees create the opportunity for a more productive company. This could also offer a competitive advantage in recruiting workers, retaining employees, and improving profit margins.

How could you help create that environment?

- SEEK BUY-IN FROM DECISION MAKERS
  Ultimately, the "boss" has to understand the value of cooperation, partnerships, and wellness. This person does not have to be a "health nut," but does have to be educated about the ramifications of an outdated, reaction-based healthcare model. Healthcare spending is just too big of a line item to ignore or not engage with. The C-suite must understand this.

- USE YOUR VOICE
  Even if you aren't a CEO or top-level decision maker—you can still make an impact. Simply begin by presenting these ideas to the coworkers or others in your circle of influence. Ideas can flow up and out just as well as they can be handed down.

- CHOOSE INSURANCE CARRIERS/BROKERS WISELY
  Insurance companies and brokers are often looked at as the enemy. In many ways, they have brought this label on themselves. Hopefully, this is beginning to shift and there's a new day dawning. Remember, your company is the customer. The brokers need your money to stay in business. You have more influence and control than you may believe. Lay out your vision for the health of your company and start working on a plan together. Your plan should save money, add value,

and improve health. If it's not doing those things, find a new partner. They work for you. Make them work.

- PARTNER WITH WELLNESS VENDORS
  Thankfully, as more companies are becoming aware of the necessity of wellness programs, more options and resources are becoming available to support these efforts. Everything from free health lectures to onsite biometric screening is available. The scale and size of your business will dictate the budget you direct toward these programs.

- EDUCATE & COMMUNICATE
  At the end of the day—for real, lasting change to happen— there is no replacement for education. The stickiness of old habits and a quick-fix culture will keep attempting to suck people out of the cooperative model. The only way to combat those forces, is through honest, authentic communication on the principles of cooperation, both physiologically and philosophically. This will be worth every minute you invest.

Corporately, it's critical to see the value of this conversation. There are ways to get involved at every level, from providing education to offering onsite vitalistic wellness clinics. One easy, affordable way to begin is by delivering very specific, personal, and effective nutritional resources straight to employees' desks.

If your company is in an urgent position right now that requires action due to rising healthcare costs, you'll want to engage in the cooperative model immediately. This is where the real savings and health promotion exist. You won't find long-term solutions by squeezing a few percentage points out of your premium.

Instead, take control by providing or partnering with people to provide a foundational understanding of health and wellness, as well as associated resources. *You* will need to champion these initiatives and support your employees/coworkers. Big Pharma and Big Insurance will not be bringing solutions to bear on this. The way out is to use less medicine and require less medical care, and this is done by promoting health activities and supporting solutions that allow a person to get the help they need.

> Most employers are involved in providing healthcare, whether directly or indirectly, so it's win–win to have healthy, productive employees to show for that investment.

We spend nearly one-third of our days at work. It's in everyone's best interest to find a way to cooperate with the body and the business to achieve the solutions everyone is seeking. The traditional medical model does not offer much to improve the well-being of employees, nor the well-being of the business.

Finding ways to integrate and support wellness and foster well-being is not a luxury; it's a necessity. It may seem easier to avoid the conversation or not get involved in your employees' wellness, and instead keep writing the check for premiums every month. But that is shortsighted and unsustainable. Make the right decision because it's right. It's time to move in a new direction. It's time to move toward cooperative wellness.

HEALTH INSURANCE WON'T KEEP YOU HEALTHY

Health insurance is the elephant in the room. In general, both employees and employers are frustrated by the expense of health insurance, but many have not yet realized they should be upset at the model, which is what's driving most of the costs. The illusion or assumption is that drugs, tests, and surgeries are the best use of the healthcare dollar—the best bang for the buck.

Many people erroneously believe (or have been convinced) that the current medical model is the best we can do. This type of thinking is embedded deeply into our culture and consciousness, which makes it difficult to explain the true gravity of this crisis. If I can adequately explain the foundational dysfunction of the health insurance model, this alone will transform both your health and pocketbook.

Health insurance is not designed to keep you healthy, it's designed to make a profit. Read that sentence again. This conflict is as disastrous as it sounds. The dysfunction of the health insurance model, coupled with handing our healthcare decisions over to bureaucrats and Wall Street, is costing us more than a few dollars—it's costing us our future.

There are many assumptions today's medical model makes that go unquestioned by consumers. We don't need more drugs, more tests, more doctors, more access, more hospitals—none of these things actually provide health. Remember, we're using more medical intervention than ever before, and we're sicker than ever.

We must stop looking to health insurance or the medical model to fix this problem. It's not designed to.

Think about your car insurance. First of all, it doesn't cover regular maintenance or non-accident-related repairs. Second, there's nothing about car insurance that prevents accidents. That's your job as the driver. There are many things that could be done to your car to make it safer, but that's up to you, not the insurance company.

The only time the insurance company usually comes into play is if there's an extensive accident. Even then, you still pay for some of the repair. Most people would rather not "use" their car insurance, because they know that can make rates go up. Healthcare tends to be the opposite. We think we should use it. We try to get our "money's worth," without realizing that we pay more for it in the end. This type of thinking and behavior fuels the problem.

We've been given this incredible human body that requires a few basic things to live and perform and heal well, but instead of doing basic maintenance, we tend to race it around, push it beyond its limits, and then expect insurance to buy us a new engine. That's not how car insurance works, and it shouldn't be how health insurance works either.

Try telling your car insurance company that you need new tires — they'll laugh at you.

Like car insurance, health insurance should exist only for traumatic, acute, or emergency situations. The rest of healthcare should be done mostly by you, outside of the walls of a hospital or pharmacy. The current medical and insurance system is more complicated than it needs to be, and it's failing to deliver improved health.

Outside-the-box insurance options do exist. There are companies that have been around for quite a while, and have operated very successfully at helping individuals and companies find unique ways to save money, incentivize healthy behaviors, and improve the healthcare experience. The model is generally called a co-op, but to the end-user it operates much like an insurance model. If you are proactive with your health, and looking to be part of the solution, this can be a great model to investigate. Some of the best are Sedera Health (for businesses) Medi-Share (for individuals).

As employees, our job is to take responsibility for our health. As employers (or leaders), we have the additional responsibility to offer access to programs and services that truly support health. One of the most exciting things about this model of cooperation is its simplicity. It's not about some complicated diet, fitness program, or expensive test.

When I was diagnosed with precancerous lesions throughout my digestive system, I was scared and confused. I believed my only option was to follow doctor's orders. The problem was, the person I was trying to learn about health from was visibly unhealthy himself and had no training in wellness or nutrition—yet I was looking to him to help get me well. Shame on me.

Remember, healthcare is our job, not our doctor's. It will never be any different. It shouldn't be.

The foods we eat, our relationships, our physical activity, and our spiritual health are the major variables that dictate our health. That is true healthcare. Sure, if you fall off a ladder and break your arm, go to the hospital—but in the meantime, take care of what the good Lord gave you.

As an employer, imagine the relief if health insurance were in the hands of your employees, for catastrophic needs. Imagine the savings. Imagine the shift in mentality this could create in the right direction—if people were spending their health dollars directly, they just might want to take better care of themselves! If you can begin to see your role as a supporter, you can begin to transform the health of your employees and the bottom line of your company.

And if you're an employee, you don't have to sit around and wait for things to change—if nothing else, you can lead by example and start carving out a healthier lifestyle any day you choose. Even if you're still "paying" into healthcare you don't use, you're still paying less in co-pays, medications, and procedures. Or if you're really passionate, you can become a vocal advocate for the things we've discussed in this book. Anyone can make a difference!

CHAPTER FIVE

The Healthcare of the Future—Today

"The doctor of the future will give no medicine, but will interest her or his patients in the care of the human frame, in a proper diet, and in the cause and prevention of disease."
— Thomas Edison

There is no downside to better understanding the body, how it heals, and how to better care for it. This understanding prevents massive amounts of disease and suffering and saves billions of dollars. The question really isn't, "Should this be the healthcare model?" but instead, "Why isn't this the healthcare model?"

After caring for thousands upon thousands of patients, I have heard every excuse under the sun as to why a person cannot engage in a holistic model of care. Each of these objections and excuses can be overcome. The reality is, you don't have the time, money, or energy *not* to consider this approach. Once the benefits of the improved healthcare model are experienced personally and collectively, people often lament that it took them so long to make the switch.

The individual, internal cooperation of the human body is already at work. You now have more awareness of the body's healing potential and capacity.

To achieve wellness and become part of the healthcare solution, you will need to engage in two ways:

- By reducing interference to the cooperation through a healthy lifestyle.
- By viewing your health and healthcare through this new vitalistic or holistic lens.

Following these two principles will help you take full responsibility for your health.

A WORD ABOUT PREVENTION

Much of what the current medical model calls prevention is actually not prevention at all. At best, it's early detection. Many times, due to the interventions suggested after the detection, or even the test itself, this process causes more harm than good.

Prevention is something that actually stops something from happening. Taking an x-ray of your teeth does nothing to prevent cavities—brushing your teeth prevents cavities. Finding cancer is much different than preventing cancer. Having a mammogram does not prevent breast cancer, but leading a healthy lifestyle does reduce risks for almost all diseases.

Let's look at some dangerous assumptions and realities regarding "preventative" testing and treatment:

- We assume the results are definitive and trust that it confirms whether we are healthy or sick. For example, you may have your cholesterol checked and be deemed "normal," but that doesn't mean you do not have heart disease, nor that your current lifestyle may not be setting you up to have heart disease! If I smoke two packs a day, and keep going to the doctor to get an x-ray of my lungs and the image continues to read all-clear—no lung tumors—should I keep smoking? On the other end, there are sometimes "false positives" with testing which have resulted in people being led to think they're sick, when they really weren't and thereby receiving unnecessary treatment (not to mention worry).

- We also assume that if we find a problem sooner, the suggested medical treatment is the best or only option. It may surprise you to learn that some breast cancers take eight to twelve years to grow large enough to be detected. So, "early" detection through testing, followed by the current protocol for breast cancer treatment, possibly could have been circumvented by changing lifestyle choices to reduce risks in the first place. Even conservative experts agree that lifestyle and environmental factors can play a significant role in increasing risk[30] (we'll discuss non-lifestyle risk factors, like genetics, in a bit).

- We must remember that the test itself has risks, the treatment has risks, and there are often many things outside of the medical model that provide much better protective results. The daily lifestyle choices we make play a larger role in prevention than expensive testing does.

The best test you can take is a lifestyle test (see resources listed in the back of this book). This is the single biggest prevention tool you can use. What this test will reveal is whether the lifestyle choices you're making are causing an increased burden on your health, thus reducing your body's ability to heal, adapt, and cooperate. This is your best chance at prevention and healing. It also saves you time, money, energy, and even stress. It allows you to be empowered and positively influence your health.

Am I suggesting that you never have these tests or procedures done? I advise you to review the research for yourself—but more importantly, carefully consider your lifestyle choices and healthcare approach during the days and years between the tests. (Personally, I do not participate in so-called preventative testing.)

Once we better understand the real odds, the real risks, the real benefits, and the main drivers of cost and saving—the real impact of caring for ourselves—it often changes our behavior. The truth will set you free.

WATCH OUT FOR SHARKS AND ALLIGATORS

We are originally from South Dakota, so when we moved to Florida, the idea of sharks and alligators was new to us. TV shows and the media can raise a big hype about these wild animals, but once you talk to the locals, they just laugh at your fear. Sure, they understand that things can happen, but it's very rare, and almost entirely preventable with a bit of awareness and some common sense. You have a much better chance of drowning in your bathtub or dying in a car accident than getting killed by a shark or alligator.

The holistic approach to healthcare takes a similar mentality. Once we understand that our best shot at health, healing, wellness, full-potential, and prevention is a matter of common sense, education, and lifestyle changes, we can move from a fear-based approach to a more positive approach.

In her book, *The Secret History of the War on Cancer,* Devra Davis describes why we're losing.[31] She exposes that we're currently aware of countless cancer-causing chemicals and lifestyle choices, yet we spend little-to-no time removing or limiting these known dangers. Instead, the cancer industry primarily focuses on finding ways to treat cancer *after* it is detected.

Type 2 diabetes, another major health concern, is now largely understood to be a disease created by lifestyle. If we continue to spend a majority of our energy and resources treating the results of our poor choices with dangerous medications, instead of working toward change, we will never solve the problem. This is as ridiculous as painting over rust on your car and thinking you've solved the problem.

When someone first explained all of this to me, it truly changed (and even saved) my life. This is one reason I'm so passionate about sharing this knowledge with anyone who will listen.

> We can't keep reacting in fear, but instead need to proactively look for ways to minimize our risk.

One important consideration we haven't touched on yet is the difference between a risk factor and a disease. For example, smoking is a risk factor for lung cancer, not the actual cause of lung cancer. I am by no means advocating smoking; I am attempting to explain the crucial difference. Smoking *increases your risk* of having lung cancer. The *cause* of lung cancer is that your body is unable to heal and adapt to the damage from smoking.

The role genetics plays in health is also important to understand. You may have specific genetic tendencies, but this does not cause cancer. Breast cancer and the BRCA gene mutations offer an example. If you inherit this mutation (risk factor), it means that you are roughly 50 percent more likely to develop breast cancer (an individual's risk may be higher or lower, based on other risk factors). A positive BRCA test result does not mean that you have (or will develop) breast cancer.[32] You may not be able to choose your genes, but you *can* have a significant influence on them, depending on the lifestyle and environment you participate in.

We are often mistakenly led to believe that a risk factor is a disease. For example, high cholesterol may be a risk factor for cardiovascular disease, but high cholesterol is not a disease in and of itself. I promise you, if there was not a class of drugs to treat high cholesterol, you would not be pushed a pill on every other commercial. Risk factors are best reduced or removed using safe, natural approaches, since drugs do not get to the cause of the risk factor.

Typically, when a risk factor is discovered to correlate to a disease, a drug is created to attempt to offset the impacts of the risk factor, which is treated as though it's a disease itself. We are then massively over-promised on the drug's benefits. The marketing gets into our heads, the fear takes over, the drugs are sold, and you think you're making the right choices for your health. You're being proactive, right?

To use the shark metaphor again, we over-emphasize and sensationalize the few shark attacks each year, creating an unbalanced hysteria. What's the answer? Selling something that maybe lowers your risk by 0.5 percent but has many potential side effects?

Would you take a pill that makes your skin taste bad to sharks but is also terrible for your body?

Crazy as this sounds (and even though the odds of a shark attack are one in 11.5 million), with the right marketing, some people just might.

YOU DO HAVE A CHOICE

Did you know that all a drug company has to prove is that the drug performs better than a placebo (or nothing)? We often assume the drug companies compare and research drugs against all of the other possible interventions and find the drug to be the best option. But this rarely, if ever, happens.

Marketing campaigns promote the assumption that drugs work far better than they actually do. If a cholesterol drug lowers cholesterol by 1 percent, it's enough to get a drug approved and marketed. Your doctor then tells you to take the drug because it lowers your cholesterol. You're led to believe that taking the drug is a life or death choice, so you choose life. But you're being misled. Drugs are marketed as if they're miracle pills. They're not.

There is another way and a better choice. The healthcare model of the future is available today. Healthy lifestyles and healthy choices lead to much better improvements than medications. Even more importantly, they do it in a way that's cooperative with the body. This is such a critical difference.

Losing weight through diet and lifestyle is very different from losing weight through drugs and surgery. The approach you take matters.

The sooner we come to the realization that drugs will not fix lifestyle problems, the sooner we can rise to a new stratosphere of healthcare. When we begin to align healthcare with a conservative approach that works with the body and places the responsibility on the patient—addressing lifestyle choices and providing support—we will have results beyond belief, and literally save trillions.

Making wise choices for yourself rather than blindly trusting your doctor might even save your life.

One disturbing study reported that "medical error" was found to be the third leading cause of death in the U.S., accounting for as many as 251,454 deaths annually.[33]

According to Martin Makary, professor of surgery at the Johns Hopkins University School of Medicine, "It boils down to people dying from the care that they receive rather than the disease for which they are seeking care."[33]

Medical error ranks well above all accidents combined, as well as respiratory disease and stroke. It's only behind cancer and heart disease. Almost unbelievable, isn't it? Another study showed that more people die from prescription drugs than all of the illegal drugs combined.[34] These findings alone demand a revolution against the current medical approach.

When people accuse me of being reckless for not taking drugs, I simply state that I'm avoiding becoming a statistic—not to mention dodging the wasted effects and expense of drugs that fail to address the cause.

There's no guarantee, folks. There's no guarantee that by taking the pills and having the tests, your disease will be prevented. The only guarantee when it comes to health is that your best bet is working with the body.

A study was done by a Harvard MD about the frequency of alternative therapy usage.[35] He was blown away to find how many people use alternative care. He assumed it was people who were uneducated and were being bamboozled by quacks. He studied the demographics and discovered the people that used alternative medicine are actually more educated. They were thinking for themselves and realized that medicine and drugs did not deliver the results they were looking for. A few years later, he conducted the study again and found even more people were turning to alternative therapy. I can only hope that the trend continues and more and more people begin looking for better solutions, better approaches to their health.

As a side note, I struggle with the term "alternative" medicine because this should be our *primary* approach. In reality, the medical model should be the alternative model. A natural, holistic, vitalistic approach is a much more logical way to approach health. Dangerous drugs and surgery should be the last-ditch effort when there is nothing left to try, and even then, used sparingly and judiciously. We have been brainwashed to believe otherwise.

We can do better. We have tried the expensive, wasteful, medical and drug approach. The results are in. It has failed to deliver on its promise.

Here's the bottom line—cooperation will never fail you. This doesn't mean you will never have a health struggle, disease, or cold, but it does mean that you have a plan and an approach to help you handle interference in the most effective way possible.

It's a new day in healthcare. It's a new day for our health individually and a new day of doing health together—cooperatively!

I believe we all want to be healthy, to not need medications or surgery, and to thrive as long as possible. If we all agree to this as our starting point, we need to stay focused on the best way to achieve that outcome. Each individual ultimately gets to make that decision for themselves and any children they care for.

As you might have noticed through this book, I am big on hammering home the overarching point that informs everything else.

Reciting truth over and again is the best way I know to get it to sink in.

I continually remind myself that the single most important variable in a person's ability to heal is their own body—that inborn, innate healing power inside them. We must never forget that's the greatest tool we have in healthcare. That is how I always approach my own health, my family's health, and my patients' health.

Our best shot at getting ourselves well is to remove as much interference as quickly as possible to allow the body to do what it's designed to do. Drugs are not a good first choice outside of an emergency situation. The cooperative model of care will lead to results that many would consider miraculous or impossible. The body is designed to heal. It wants to be well. Health is not an accident or chance.

Although you probably were not expecting me to share a poem with you, I cannot think of a more fitting way to wrap things up. The sentiments of this poem are perhaps even more reflective of our culture today—with all of our "advances," have we really progressed at all since this poem was written in 1895?

May we wake up and evolve out of the outdated, rescue mentality of chemical-based healthcare and into a new paradigm of cooperative wellness that works with the inborn wisdom of the body, and the grace found within, to protect our gift of health.

It is ours to lose or sustain.

"THE AMBULANCE AT THE BOTTOM OF THE HILL"
By Joseph Mullins

'Twas a dangerous cliff, as they freely confessed,
Though to walk near its crest was so pleasant;
But over its terrible edge there had slipped
A duke and full many a peasant.

So the people said something would have to be done,
But their projects did not at all tally;
Some said, "Put a fence 'round the edge of the cliff,"
Some, "An ambulance down in the valley."

But the cry for the ambulance carried the day,
For it spread through the neighboring city;
A fence may be useful or not, it is true,
But each heart became full of pity.

For those who slipped over the dangerous cliff;
And the dwellers in highway and alley
Gave pounds and gave pence, not to put up a fence,
But an ambulance down in the valley.
"For the cliff is all right, if you're careful," they said,

"And, if folks even slip and are dropping,
It isn't the slipping that hurts them so much
As the shock down below when they're stopping."

So day after day, as these mishaps occurred,
Quick forth would those rescuers sally
To pick up the victims who fell off the cliff,
With their ambulance down in the valley.

Then an old sage remarked: "It's a marvel to me
That people give far more attention
To repairing results than to stopping the cause,
When they'd much better aim at prevention.

Let us stop at its source all this mischief," cried he,
"Come, neighbors and friends, let us rally;
If the cliff we will fence, we might almost dispense
With the ambulance down in the valley."

"Oh he's a fanatic," the others rejoined,
"Dispense with the ambulance? Never!
He'd dispense with all charities, too, if he could;
No! No! We'll support them forever.

Aren't we picking up folks just as fast as they fall?
And shall this man dictate to us? Shall he?
Why should people of sense stop to put up a fence,
While the ambulance works in the valley?"

But the sensible few, who are practical too,

Will not bear with such nonsense much longer;
They believe that prevention is better than cure,
And their party will soon be the stronger.

Encourage them then, with your purse, voice, and pen,
And while other philanthropists dally,
They will scorn all pretense, and put up a stout fence
On the cliff that hangs over the valley.

Better guide well the young than reclaim them when old,
For the voice of true wisdom is calling.
"To rescue the fallen is good, but 'tis best
To prevent other people from falling."

Better close up the source of temptation and crime
Than deliver from dungeon or galley;
Better put a strong fence 'round the top of the cliff
Than an ambulance down in the valley.

AFTERWORD

Life without Fear

"Never underestimate the power of a small group of committed people to change the world. In fact, it is the only thing that ever has." — Margaret Mead

I would suggest that the opposite of fear is hope, or faith. This book is intended to provide hope. One of the most powerful aspects of health, healing, or moving forward in any area of life is hope—to believe that things can be better, or different.

But we often think that hope is on par with wishful thinking. I disagree. Hope is not simply saying, "I hope I feel better." True hope is based on understanding. You can now have a more determined hope because you understand that the body is so magnificently designed to heal. Hope is akin to the word faith, which is often discounted too quickly due to cultural context—yet I am compelled to include it. After all, even someone who says they have faith in nothing, has come to that conclusion based on something. Sometimes we assign faith without even realizing it.

For instance, many have put their faith in the medical model simply because it's all they know, even though that faith is largely unfounded. Shouldn't we instead invest our faith in something that has the most likely chance of being the most helpful?

Oddly, we don't usually look at it that way. We don't view taking drugs and relying on invasive testing and dangerous surgery as relating to faith or hope, when in fact that's exactly what it is, even if it doesn't consciously feel that way. Often it's because you don't have enough information to make an informed decision, so you trust someone you believe has more information than you do.

Imagine if your doctor told you the full truth about the risks verses benefits of a medical intervention, and also made you aware of other options that are known to be safe and helpful—which option would you put your faith in?

Having faith doesn't mean you absolutely know—without a single doubt—that something will or won't happen (or is/isn't true). It means you believe that this is the best option (or carries the greatest possibility of truth). Even if you don't think much about it one way or the other, if you simply go with the flow—by default, you're placing your faith in that current.

Reading *Life without Fear,* by Dr. Fred Barge,[36] changed my life. There are many layers to that title, but as it relates to cooperation, here is the wisdom within: There is profound peace once you understand cooperation and focus on improving it.

Instead of being afraid of catching a cold, or getting cancer or Alzheimer's, you can remember this simple but profound concept.

The body is masterful at cooperation. When a body—or a company, or a family, or a soccer team—is cooperating, it has its best chance at success. Period. Guaranteed. The better it's cooperating, the better the outcome every time. It follows that we must shift our focus to that one thing—improving cooperation—by either removing barriers or providing resources. We don't have to live in fear anymore about our health.

The future is bright if we are willing to open the door and walk through. Step by step, this can be accomplished with all of us working together, cooperatively.

"All things work together for the good of those who believe."
— *Romans 8:28, paraphrase*

NOTES

1. "Exploring the Harmful Effects of Health Care," Charles M. Kilo MD MPH, Eric B. Larson MD MPH, *The Journal of the American Medical Association,* July 2009, http://jama.jamanetwork.com/article.aspx?articleid=184158.

2. "Questioning the Benefits of Statins," Eddie Vos, Colin P. Rose, *CMAJ,* November 2005, http://www.cmaj.ca/content/173/10/1207.2.full.

3. "Self-Insurance on Steroids," Bruce Shutan, *The Self-Insurer,* August 2014, http://www.bruceshutan.com/uploads/3/4/4/2/3442746/self-insurance_ on_steroids.pdf.

4. "U.S. Healthcare Spending On Track To Hit $10,000 Per Person This Year," Dan Munro, *Forbes,* January 2015, http://www.forbes.com/sites/ danmunro/2015/01/04/u-s-healthcare-spending-on-track-to-hit-10000-per- person-this-year/#1c6351ef294c.

5. "Carol Dweck," *Wikipedia,* accessed August 2016, https://en.wikipedia. org/wiki/Carol_Dweck.

6. "It's True: Drug Companies Are Bombarding Your TV with More Ads Than Ever," Jason Millman, *The Washington Post,* March 2015, https://www.washingtonpost.com/news/wonk/wp/2015/03/23/ yes-drug-companies-are-bombarding-your-tv-with-more-ads-than-ever.

7. "Labour of love: The demise of Traditional Midwifery," Matilda Lee, *Ecologist,* March 2012, http://www.theecologist.org/News/news_analysis/1272162/ labour_of_love_the_demise_of_traditional_midwifery.html.

8. "A Randomized Trial of Vertebroplasty for Painful Osteoporotic Vertebral Fractures," Rachelle Buchbinder PhD, Richard H. Osborne PhD, Peter R. Ebeling MD, et al., *The New England Journal of Medicine,* August 2009, http://www.nejm.org/doi/full/10.1056/NEJMoa0900429#t=article.

9. "Affect and Emotion: A New Social Science Understanding," Margaret Wetherell, *Google Books,* 63, https://books.google.com/books?id=4Ci0hIQu K3oC&pg=PA63&lpg=PA63#v=onepage&q&f=false.

10. "One Cigarette Takes 14 Minutes of Your Life," *Healthlab,* October 2014, https://www.healthlab.tv/news/6569_one-cigarette-takes-14-minutes-of-your-life.html.

11. "Back Surgery: Too Many, Too Costly and Too Ineffective," *To Your Health,* J.C. Smith, June 2011, http://www.toyourhealth.com/mpacms/tyh/article. php?id=1447.

12. "Long-Term Follow-up of a Randomized Clinical Trial Assessing the Efficacy of Medication, Acupuncture, and Spinal Manipulation for Chronic Mechanical Spinal Pain Syndromes," Reinhold Muller PhD, Lynton G.F. Giles DC PhD, *Journal of Manipulative and Physiological Therapeutics,* January 2005, http://www.danmurphydc.com/wordpress/ wp-content/uploads/archive/2004/Article_34-04.muller.pdf.

13. "Biohack Your Acid Reflux: Treatment Without Dangerous Drugs," Dr. Kevin Passero, accessed August 2016, https://www.bulletproofexec.com/ acid-reflux-treatment-diet-without-drugs.

14. "Rocks in Your Backpack," Dr. James Chestnut, *YouTube,* March 2011, https://www.youtube.com/watch?v=xw8lyZwI298.

15. "Nearly 60 Percent of Americans — the Highest Ever — Are Taking Prescription Drugs," Brady Dennis, *The Washington Post,* November 2015, https://www.washingtonpost.com/news/to-your-health/wp/2015/11/03/ more-americans-than-ever-are-taking-prescription-drugs.

16. "So Young and So Many Pills," Anna Wilde Mathews, *The Wall Street Journal,* December 2010, http://www.wsj.com/articles/SB1000142405297 0203731004576046073896475588.

17. "Prescription Thugs: New Documentary Shows Big Pharma's Role in Addiction and Tragedy," Amy Dresner, *The Fix,* January 2016, https:// www.thefix.com/prescription-thugs-new-documentary-shows-big-pharmas-role-addiction-and-tragedy.

18. "So Inherently Dangerous that Only Two Countries in the World Have Legalized This and the U.S. Is One of Them," *Mercola.com,* July 2012, http://articles.mercola.com/sites/articles/archive/2012/07/16/drug-companies-ads-dangers.aspx.

19. "Comic books. Lesson plans. How Drug Companies Target Kids," Rebecca Robbins, *STAT,* June 2016, https://www.statnews.com/2016/06/02/drug-marketing-kids.

20. "2015 Annual Report, International Comparisons," *America's Health Rankings,* accessed August 2016, http://www.americashealthrankings.org/reports/annual.

21. "Why Do Americans Consume 80 Percent Of All Prescription Painkillers?," Tyler Durden, *Zero Hedge,* March 2016, http://www.zerohedge.com/news/2016-03-15/why-do-americans-consume-80-percent-all-prescription-painkillers.

22. "Vioxx Lawsuit," *Drugwatch,* accessed August 2016, https://www.drugwatch.com/vioxx/lawsuit.

23. "Why Are Nearly a Third of Childbirths Cesareans?," *Mercola.com,* June 2009, http://articles.mercola.com/sites/articles/archive/2009/06/04/why-are-nearly-a-third-of-childbirths-cesareans.aspx.

24. "Study: 71% of ED Visits Unnecessary, Avoidable," Sabrina Rodak, *Becker's Hospital Review,* April 2013, http://www.beckershospitalreview.com/patient-flow/study-71-of-ed-visits-unnecessary-avoidable.html.

25. "Your Greatest Weapon Against Breast Cancer (Not Mammograms)," *Mercola.com,* March 2012, http://articles.mercola.com/sites/articles/archive/2012/03/03/experts-say-avoid-mammograms.aspx.

26. "Do you really need a yearly physical exam?," *CBS News,* January 2015, http://www.cbsnews.com/news/do-you-really-need-a-yearly-physical-exam.

27. "Death by Medicine, Part I," Gary Null PhD, Carolyn Dean MD ND, Martin Feldman MD, et al., *Mercola.com,* November 2003, http://articles.mercola.com/sites/articles/archive/2003/11/26/death-by-medicine-part-one.aspx.

28. *Network* (1976) Quotes, *IMDb,* accessed August 2016, http://www.imdb.com/title/tt0074958/quotes.

29. "Mayo Clinic Chief: U.S. Health Care System 'Doomed,'" *Daily Kos,* May 2006, http://www.dailykos.com/story/2006/5/2/206751/-.

30. "Environmental Risk Factors," Laurie Wertich, *Cancer Treatment Centers of America,* accessed August 2016, http://www.cancercenter.com/community/thrive/environmental-risk-factors.

31. Devra Davis, *The Secret History of the War on Cancer,* (Basic Books, 2007).

32. "BRCA1 and BRCA2: Cancer Risk and Genetic Testing," *National Cancer Institute,* accessed August 2016, http://www.cancer.gov/about-cancer/causes-prevention/genetics/brca-fact-sheet#q2.

33. "Researchers: Medical Errors Now Third Leading Cause of Death in United States," Ariana Eunjung Cha, *The Washington Post,* May 2016, https://www.washingtonpost.com/news/to-your-health/wp/2016/05/03/researchers-medical-errors-now-third-leading-cause-of-death-in-united-states.

34. "Prescription Drugs Are More Deadly Than Street Drugs," Scott A. Bonn PhD, *Psychology Today,* April 28, 2014, https://www.psychologytoday.com/blog/wicked-deeds/201404/prescription-drugs-are-more-deadly-street-drugs.

35. "Trends in Alternative Medicine Use in the United States," David M. Eisenberg MD, et al., *The Journal of the American Medical Association,* November 1998, http://jama.jamanetwork.com/article.aspx?articleid=188148.

36. F. H. Barge, *Life Without Fear,* (Bawden Bros, 2001).

RESOURCES

A wellness-based health risk assessment:
https://apps.bluezones.com/vitality

Follow the ongoing conversation:
https://drbenrall.wordpress.com

Individual and corporate supplements:
www.achievenutrition.com

A unique benefit design:
www.ioausa.com

Fitness:
http://intrvlburn.com

Online streaming of the ultimate Source of wellness:
www.firstorlando.com

Interested in becoming a wellness practitioner?
www.life.edu

Learn to live on purpose:
http://on-purpose.com/start

www.ingramcontent.com/pod-product-compliance
Lightning Source LLC
Chambersburg PA
CBHW070119290526
45789CB00005B/2076